NURSE'S CLINICAL POCKET MANUAL:
NURSING DIAGNOSES, CARE PLANNING, AND DOCUMENTATION

Mary Frances Moorhouse, R.N., CCP, CCRN, CRRN

Nurse Consultant
TNT-RN Enterprises and Fortis Corporation
Colorado Springs, Colorado

and

Marilynn E. Doenges, B.S.N., M.A., C.S.

Clinical Specialist
Adult Psychiatric/Mental Health Nursing
Private Practice
Colorado Springs, Colorado

Copyright © 1990 by F. A. Davis Company

All rights reserved. This book is protected by copyright. No part of it may be reproduced, stored in a retrieval system, or transmitted in any form or by any means, electronic, mechanical, photocopying, recording, or otherwise, without written permission from the publisher.

Printed in the United States of America
Last digit indicates print number: 10 9 8 7 6 5 4 3 2 1

Authorization to photocopy items for internal or personal use, or the internal or personal use of specific clients, is granted by F. A. Davis Company for users registered with the Copyright Clearance Center (CCC) Transactional Reporting Service, provided that the fee of $.10 per copy is paid directly to CCC, 27 Congress St., Salem, MA 01970. For those organizations that have been granted a photocopy license by CCC, a separate system of payment has been arranged. The fee code for users of the Transactional Reporting Service is: 8036-6314/90 0 + $.10.

Library of Congress Cataloging-in-Publication Data

Moorhouse, Mary Frances, 1947-
Nurse's clinical pocket manual.

Includes bibliographical references.
1. Nursing assessment--Handbooks, manuals, etc.
2. Physical diagnosis--Handbooks, manuals, etc.
3. Nursing care plans--Handbooks, manuals, etc.
I. Doenges, Marilynn E., 1922- . II. Title.
[DNLM: 1. Medical Records--handbooks. 2. Nursing Assessment--methods--handbooks. 3. Patient Care Planning--handbooks. WY 39 M825n]
RT48.M66 1990 610.73 90-2934
ISBN 0-8036-6314-5

DEDICATION

This book is dedicated:

- to all the nurses (students and instructors, staff nurses and administrators, nurse practitioners, clinical specialists) who have been struggling to put it together.
- to our families, who continue to support us in so many ways, our love and thanks.
- to Robert Martone, Senior Editor, who was instrumental in helping us develop and refine this work.
- to Alan Sorkowitz, Nursing Developmental Editor; Ruth DE George, Executive Secretary/Editorial; and Nancee Vogel, Production Editor, who assisted in the production of this book.

PREFACE

This helpful guide focuses on care plan formulation, documentation, and charting tips. Included are sample assessment tools and prototype care plans to help nurses learn to develop their care planning skills.

Section I contains a brief review in Chapter 1 of the theories and models of nursing to help the nurse understand the direction in which nursing is moving to determine the philosophic basis of the profession. Chapters 2 and 3 discuss the nursing process with a section on data collection and a nursing assessment tool designed to help the nurse identify appropriate nursing diagnoses. Chapter 4 discusses how to construct a care plan using nursing diagnoses, and documentation of care is addressed in Chapter 5.

Section II presents seven prototype care plans (case studies) that have been formulated to demonstrate application of nursing process (data collection, problem identification, planning, implementation, and evaluation) and that represent a variety of health care settings.

Section III provides selected nursing diagnostic statements for approximately 300 disorders/health problems reflecting all specialty areas.

The practicing nurse as well as the student will find this handy reference guide indispensable for facilitating the assessment and diagnosis steps of the nursing process and simplifying and maintaining quality for their documentation process.

ACKNOWLEDGEMENTS

A special thanks to our friends and colleagues who read and critiqued the manuscript.

Linda J. Brown, R.N., B.S.
Director of Quality Assurance and Managed Care
Cedar Springs, Psychiatric Hospital
Colorado Springs, Colorado

Jacqueline Fawcett, Ph.D., F.A.A.N.
Associate Professor
University of Pennsylvania
School of Nursing
Philadelphia, Pennsylvania

Alice Geissler, R.N., CCRN
Contract Practitioner
Critical Care
Colorado Springs, Colorado

Betty Hopping, Ph.D., R.N.
Dean and CEO
Beth-El College of Nursing
Colorado Springs, Colorado

Finis Nabors
Director of Staff Development
Oaks Treatment Center
Austin, Texas

CONTENTS

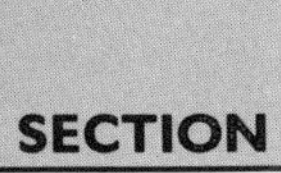

SECTION I

FOUNDATIONS OF CLINICAL PRACTICE

This section contains an introduction to nursing theories and conceptual models outlining the philosophic basis of the profession. The use of nursing process and diagnosis to identify patient needs and goals of care is presented. Additional chapters expand the steps of the nursing process as visualized through the creation of the plan of care. Finally, the vital role of documentation is discussed in detail to facilitate the recording of nursing activities and patient response.

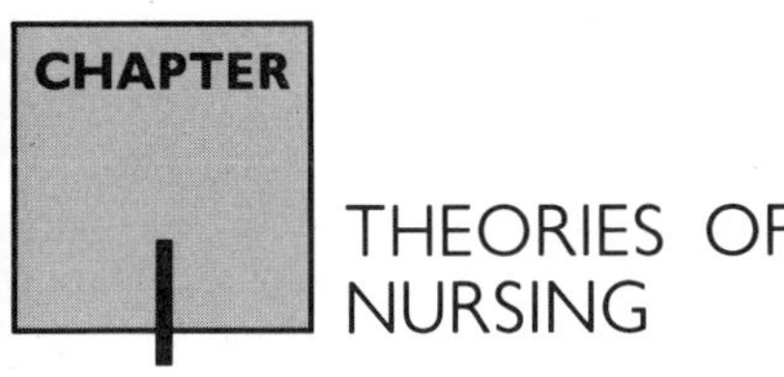

CHAPTER 1 THEORIES OF NURSING

The American Nurses Association (1980) *Social Policy Statement* declared that "An occupation becomes a profession when its practitioners use scientific knowledge to understand and to treat the phenomena within its socially delegated domain (of) service." Nursing has struggled with its image, and although it is called a "profession", the attempt to define the realm of practice has led in many different directions. Some of these directions have been identified by nurse theorists in an attempt to provide nurses with an understanding of their profession and as a basis for practice.

The phenomena of particular interest to the nursing profession are the person, the environment (internal and external), health, and nursing (Fawcett, 1989). Person refers to the recipient of nursing care, including individuals, families, communities, and other groups. The environment refers to the care recipient's significant others and physical surroundings as well as the setting in which nursing care occurs. Health is the care recipient's state of well-being, which can range from high-level wellness to terminal illness. Nursing refers to the actions taken by nurses on behalf of or in conjunction with recipients of care, directed toward maintaining, modifying, or somehow managing the current health state. The nursing actions typically are viewed as a systematic process of assessment, diagnosis, planning, intervention, and evaluation.

Scientific knowledge about these phenomena is

codified in nursing's abstract and general conceptual models and in nursing's more specific and concrete theories. Each conceptual model or theory presents a distinctive lens through which the person, the environment, health, and nursing actions are viewed. More specifically, conceptual models and theories provide various guidelines for nursing practice through articulation of a systematic nursing process, including a format for assessment, a taxonomy of nursing diagnosis, a planning strategy, a typology of nursing interventions, and criteria for evaluation of the effects of nursing care.

The following overviews of several conceptual models of nursing and nursing theories are presented to illustrate the diversity of nursing process guidelines for the practicing nurse and student. The distinction between conceptual models and theories is the level of abstraction. However, most theories deal with only a part of the whole process of patient care; for instance Orlando's theory deals only with the interpersonal process between nurse and patient.

AQUILERA AND MESSICK'S THEORY OF CRISIS INTERVENTION

Major Focus

This theory considers crisis a stressful event or change in the individual's life, involving a loss or threat of loss that disrupts the individual's equilibrium. Several behavioral theories have been synthesized in the development of this theory. Three balancing factors—realistic perception of the event, situational supports, and coping mechanisms—are needed to maintain equilibrium and avoid a crisis.

Goal of Nursing

The nursing goal identified by Aquilera and Messick is to avert or reduce the risk of a crisis and maintain equilibrium.

Nursing Process Format

This theory uses all components of the nursing process and is applicable in planning nursing implementation strategies.

HALL'S CONCEPTUAL MODEL

Major Focus

This model describes nursing as consisting of care (activities of daily living), core (changes in health status and their effects on lifestyle), and cure. These concepts are interrelated and are depicted as three interlocking circles that meet the physical, emotional, and interactive needs of the patient.

Goal of Nursing

The nurse's role is the therapeutic use of self, and s/he functions independently to meet the care and core aspects and interdependently with other health team members in the cure component.

Nursing Process Format

This theory follows the nursing process, that is, assessment, problem identification, planning, intervention, and evaluation.

JOHNSON'S BEHAVIORAL SYSTEMS MODEL

Major Focus

Dorothy Johnson's model is a synthesis of theories and concepts from the behavioral and biologic sciences that are integrated into a systems framework. Johnson also has applied theories of stress and adaptation in this model. It is based on the interaction and pattern of the behavioral system and seven subsystems. These are linked and open, and a disturbance in one is likely to affect the other. These subsystems are defined as follows:

- *Attachment or affiliative:* To relate to or belong to something or someone.
- *Ingestive:* To take in from the environment needed resources to maintain integrity, achieve pleasure, or internalize the external environment.
- *Eliminative:* To expel biologic waste from the system.
- *Dependency:* To obtain resources needed for assistance, attention, reassurance, and security (aids in gaining approval, attention, trust, and reliance).
- *Sexual:* Procreation and gratification at feeling attractive to and cared about by others.
- *Aggressive:* Protection of oneself and others from potentially threatening objects, persons, or ideas (self-preservation mechanism).
- *Achievement:* To master or control oneself or one's environment through seeking some standard of excellence, such as physical, social, or creative skills.

Goal of Nursing

According to Johnson, the goal of nursing is "to restore, maintain, or attain behavioral system balance and stability at the highest possible level for the individual." The goal may be expanded to include helping the person achieve a more optimal level of balance and functioning.

Nursing Process Format

Although Johnson's model does not identify a specific nursing process, it does document utility in practice, administration, and research and has provided direction for curriculum development. It is applicable to the individual in the nursing process, and the nurse is expected to base judgments on an explicit value system.

KING'S INTERACTING SYSTEMS MODEL

Major Focus

This conceptual model is based on the assumption that the focus of nursing is an open system of human beings interacting with their environment, leading to a state of health for individuals, which is an ability to function in social roles.

Goals of Nursing

Nursing is defined by King as a process of action, reaction, and interaction between patient and nurse. The goal is to help individuals and groups attain, maintain, and restore health or, when this is not possible, to help the individual die with dignity.

Nursing Process Format

King believes that nursing is practiced through the nursing process, which is defined as a dynamic, ongoing interpersonal process. Patient and nurse are viewed as a system with an emphasis on patient participation, including mutual goal setting and exploration of means to achieve those goals. The components are identified as action, reaction, interaction, and transaction.

LEVINE'S CONSERVATION MODEL

Major Focus

This model is focused on the theoretic basis for nurses' actions with scientific concepts underlying nursing processes. The model is developed from the basic assumption that nursing intervention is a conservation activity. The holistic nature of the human response to the environment provides the rationale for substantive principles of nursing. This model focuses on the individual person, who is described as a holistic being. The internal and external environment are identified, and health and disease are characterized as patterns of adaptive change.

Goal of Nursing

This model promotes wholeness for all people, well or sick, and provides nursing with a logically congruent, holistic view of the person and an effective guide for nursing actions.

Nursing Process Format

Levine believes that nursing processes are derived from scientific knowledge. Conservation is defined as a "keeping together" function, and, although an explicit nursing process is not identified, the components of assessment and identification of nursing care needs are discussed. Levine also refers to nursing diagnosis as a "diagnosis of disease made by a nurse." Identification of nursing care needs is called *trophicognosis*, which she defines as "a nursing care judgment arrived at by the scientific method."

NEUMAN'S (HEALTH-CARE) SYSTEMS MODEL

Major Focus

This model is also based on systems theory as well as on Selye's theory of stress, adaptation theories, and holistic approaches to individuals and health care. The occurrence of stressors, the reaction of the patient to the stressors, and the patient's physiologic, psychologic, sociocultural, and developmental status are considered. The model is seen as a comprehensive holistic view of the patient system.

Goal of Nursing

Neuman's model facilitates optimal wellness for the patient through retention, attainment, or maintenance of patient system stability and assists the patient in creating and shaping reality in a desired direction through purposeful interventions.

Nursing Process Format

According to Neuman, nursing process encompasses three steps or categories: nursing diagnosis, nursing goals, and nursing outcomes. The patient is an active participant in the process, and systems thinking is reflected. Both systems thinking and nursing actions are purposeful and goal-directed.

OREM'S SELF-CARE FRAMEWORK

Major Focus

Initially, the need for organizing a framework for nursing knowledge and the need to identify what are specifically nursing problems led to the formulation of Orem's conceptual framework. This theory reflects the belief that self-care activities are the actions that the patient undertakes to maintain his/her well-being. The nurse becomes "another self" when the judgment has been made that an individual should be receiving nursing care. The idea that human beings can benefit from nursing when they have health-derived or health-related limitations that prevent them from engaging in continued self-care or care of dependent others is the basis for this theory. Orem's self-care framework is classified as a developmental model with characteristics of growth, development, and maturation addressed by the developmental self-care requisites and by the consideration of self-care agency adjusted for age and developmental state.

Goal of Nursing

As defined by Orem, the nurses role is to help people meet their own therapeutic self-care demands. This goal is comprised of the following three components: (1) helping the patient to accomplish therapeutic self-care, (2) helping the patient move toward responsible self-care action, and (3) helping members of the patient's family or other person become competent in providing and managing the patient's care using appropriate nursing supervision and consultation.

Nursing Process Format

The nursing process is presented in the following three steps: (1) diagnosis and prescription; (2) designing and planning; and (3) producing care to regulate therapeutic self-care demand and self-care agency.

ORLANDO'S THEORY

Major Focus

The major concepts in this theory propose that (1) the function of professional nursing is to discover and meet the patient's immediate needs for help; (2) the product of professional nursing is improvement in the immediate verbal and nonverbal behavior of the patient; and (3) the presenting behavior of the patient, regardless of the form in which it appears, may be a plea for help.

Goal of Nursing

In this theory, the role of the nurse is to discover and meet the patient's immediate needs for help.

Nursing Process Format

The nursing process is the basis for nursing action, and the nurse is accountable for his/her behavior. The nurse must identify the problems in a disciplined way, expressing them as a question to ensure that the perceptions are correct. Thus the process enables the nurse to discover and meet the patient's immediate need for help. It is important to avoid making decisions for others. Therefore, the nurse's role is to assist people in making their own decisions, including the consequences and potential for affecting future decisions.

ROGER'S SCIENCE OF UNITARY HUMAN BEINGS

Major Focus

Martha Rogers also developed her conceptual system from a realization that there was a need for an organized body of nursing knowledge. She was a pioneer in the development of unique nursing knowledge, identifying the central phenomenon of interest to the discipline of nursing as man. She has focused attention to the environment as an equally important phenomenon for study.

This conceptual system is viewed as a science of unitary human beings with the education and practice directed toward the maintenance and promotion of health, prevention of illness, and care and rehabilitation of the sick and disabled. Greater knowledge of these concepts is required to use Rogers' framework.

Goal of Nursing

The goal is predicated on a view of the practitioner as "an environmental component for the individual receiving services." It focuses on promotion of health and the integral relationship between the human and environmental energy fields.

Nursing Process Format

Nursing process follows from the science of nursing and focuses on the person as a unified whole with a need for individualized nursing care. Interventions must be personalized, based on the needs of the individual. Rogers regards the nursing process as a modality for implementation of nursing knowledge but lacking in any substance of its own. She has not identified a particular nursing process format, but mentions assessment, diagnosis, goal setting, intervention, and evaluation.

ROY'S ADAPTATION MODEL

Major Focus

In Sister Callista Roy's model, the focus of nursing is the person, although the model also may be applied to a family, a community, or society. The recipient of nursing care is identified as an adaptive system that may or may not be adapting positively. Roy identified the biologic, psychologic, and social components within the context of the totality of the person. The four adaptive modes are (1) physiologic, (2) self-concept, (3) role function, and (4) interdependence.

Goal of Nursing

Nursing's goal is to promote adaptation in each of the adaptive modes, in situations of health and illness. Roy values the active participation of patients in their nursing care when they are able to do so.

Nursing Process Format

This model involves a detailed nursing process defined as a problem-solving procedure for gathering data, identifying problems, selecting and implementing approaches, and evaluating results in relation to care of the ill or potentially ill person. The following six steps are identified: assessment of behaviors, assessment of influencing factors (stimuli), nursing diagnosis, goal setting, selection of intervention approaches, and evaluation.

WATSON'S THEORY OF HUMAN CARE

Major Focus

The primary subject matter of Jean Watson's theory includes (1) nursing within a human science and art context; (2) a mutuality of person/self of both nurse and patient with mind-body-gestalt within a context of intersubjectivity; and (3) human care relationship in nursing as a moral ideal that includes concepts such as phenomenal field, actual caring occasion, and transpersonal caring. The notions of health/illness and environment/universe and how they interact, transact, and transcend the physical-material objects and values of life are inherent in this model.

Goal of Nursing

According to Watson, the goal of nursing is to help persons "gain a higher degree of harmony within the mind, body, and soul which generates self-knowledge, self-reverence, self-healing, and self-care process while allowing increasing diversity."

Professional nurses systematically employ the scientific problem-solving method to help with decision making in all nursing situations. Facilitating learning to improve the accuracy and realism of a person's perceptions about health care concerns is also seen as a goal of nursing.

Nursing Process Format

Nursing process must be practiced as a part of scientific problem solving. Concepts/interventions have been developed that are referred to as *carative* factors, which are the factors that the nurse uses in the delivery of health care to the patient such as formation of a humanistic-altruistic system of values, instillation of faith-hope, and cultivation of sensitivity to self and others. All other carative factors depend on the development of these three.

CONCLUSION

A major issue in the discussion of the theoretic basis of nursing is the need for several different perspectives versus the need for a single unified approach to nursing. At this time, there is limited experience with conceptual models and theories and it is impossible to know which parts of which models and theories most profitably could be included in a unified model or in a combination of a few models and theories. The danger in excluding any ideas at this time is that important ideas might be lost. It seems that competition of multiple models and theories is needed to determine the superiority of one or more. This issue can only be resolved when many nurses have worked enough with all of the models and theories to know which of them leads to problems and solutions that are deemed significant for nursing.

The various models/theories need to be tested further, refined, and made understandable and available so that nursing can base its practice on a sound, scientific grounding. As nurses learn and begin to incorporate an explicit model or theory of nursing into their practice, they will understand the function of nursing and become more responsible and accountable to their patients and in interactions with other team members.

Regardless of the framework chosen, the nurse must assess the patient to determine individual needs, then the plan of care the nurse develops to meet these needs must be recorded and evaluated to promote continuity of care in a timely manner. This can be accomplished through the construction of a written plan of care reflecting this nursing process.

CHAPTER 2

NURSING PROCESS AND NURSING DIAGNOSIS

There is a growing awareness that nursing care is a key factor in patient survival and in the maintenance, rehabilitative, and preventive aspects of health care. Publication of both the American Nurses Association (ANA) *Social Policy Statement* (1980), which defines nursing as the diagnosis and treatment of human responses to actual and potential health problems, and the ANA *Standards of Practice* have provided impetus and support for the use of nursing diagnosis in the practice setting. Changes in the health-care system such as prospective payment plans and movement out of the acute care (hospital) to other settings (e.g., long-term/convalescent, rehabilitation, home health services) accentuate the need for a common framework of communication and documentation. This would promote continuity of care for the patient who moves from one area of the health-care system to another.

With the "knowledge explosion" that began in the late 1950s, many disciplines have expanded their horizons. Nursing is no exception, having accepted the concept of total, individualized care of patients as a basis for effective, therapeutic nursing care. Philosophically, this has been termed a holistic approach to health care. In implementing the concept, the nursing profession has identified a process that contributes to the prevention of illness as well as to the restoration and maintenance of health. Nursing process is adapted from the scientific approach to problem solving and requires the skills of (1) assessment (systematic collection of data relating to patients and their problems/needs); (2) problem identification (interpretation of data); (3) planning (choice of solutions); (4) implementation (putting the plan into action); and (5) evaluation (assessing the effectiveness of the plan and changing the plan as indicated by the current needs). While nurses use these terms separately, in reality they are not linear but interrelated, forming a continuous circle of thought and action. Thus, they provide an efficient method of organizing thought processes for clinical decision making (Fig. 2–1). Whether the nurse recognizes this process, s/he uses the steps, at least mentally, from the moment a patient is admitted through to discharge. For example:

A 15-year-old girl complains of difficulty breathing after being admitted for a recurrent asthma attack. The nurse assesses the patient's vital signs,

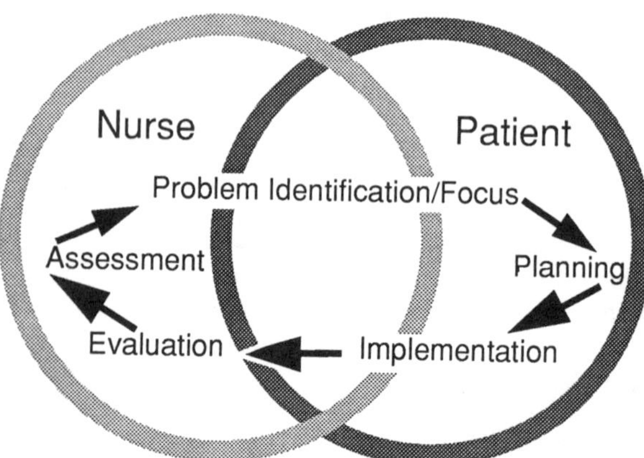

Figure 2–1. Nursing process continuum for clinical decision making.

auscultates her lungs, and notes respiratory depth and presence of cyanosis/dyspnea. S/he then reviews the patient orders for prn therapy (assessment). The nurse concludes that the patient is experiencing ineffective airway clearance related to bronchial muscle spasm and retained secretions (problem identification/focus). The nurse decides to use a prn inhaler and to encourage the patient to use pursed-lip breathing and relaxation techniques (plan). S/he assists the patient in the use of the inhaler as prescribed, then demonstrates techniques to help the patient regain control of respirations (implementation). Ten minutes later, the patient's respiratory rate is decreased, depth increased, and the skin/mucous membrane color is pale pink. The patient appears relaxed and reports that her breathing has eased (evaluation).

The nursing-care system that emerges is recognized as containing "nursing's body of knowledge" and is to be shared with other health-care professionals in order to provide comprehensive patient care. There are overlapping areas of responsibility for assessment, diagnosis, delivery, and documentation of care within the health team.

The critical element for effective, therapeutic nursing care is thorough, appropriately performed assessments. Understanding the individuality of care requires the integration of a personal, sociologic, psychologic, and medical history with a physical examination and results of diagnostic studies. Looking at the data as a whole provides the nurse with a comprehensive picture of the patient from which to identify problems/concerns. Individual responses to these concerns then lead to nursing diagnoses and formulation of a patient problem statement/focus.

The nursing diagnosis labels identified by the North American Nursing Diagnosis Association (NANDA) provide a framework for using the nursing process (Table 2–1). While there are differing definitions of nursing diagnosis, we have chosen to use Shoemaker's, taken from the *Classification of Nursing Diagnosis: Proceedings of the Fifth National Conference.* (Kim et al, 1984). "Nursing diagnosis is a clinical judgment about an individual, family or community which is derived through a deliberate, systematic process of data collection and analysis. It provides the basis for prescriptions for definitive therapy for which the nurse is accountable. It is expressed concisely and it includes the etiology of the condition when known."

The responsibility for establishing the nursing diagnosis varies according to the organizational framework of nursing-care delivery used by the particular service organization (e.g., functional method, team method, primary care, and case method). Although nursing practice is more than nursing diagnosis, it provides a common language for identifying patient problems, nursing interventions, and evaluation tools.

Nurses may feel at risk in committing themselves to documenting a nursing diagnosis. However, the nursing diagnosis is only as good as the information currently available, and there are many resources that can assist in identifying and formulating the problem statement. Unlike medical diagnoses, nursing diagnoses change as the patient progresses through various stages of illness/maladaption to problem resolution. It is important to note that the medical diagnosis may suggest nursing diagnoses, but that the two are not synonymous. As nurses begin to use nursing diagnoses on a daily basis, they will become more comfortable and familiar with the value of the diagnoses in the communication process.

We believe that any nursing diagnosis can be actual or potential, and although this issue has not been formally resolved by NANDA, it has been used in this manner in this book. Recognizing that the current NANDA list of diagnostic labels is not comprehensive, nurses need to become familiar with these parameters and validate their usefulness. As noted in Table 2–1, we present recommendations as formulated through the Eighth NANDA Conference. Brackets indicate additions/changes that we have made to clarify or enhance the accepted nursing diagnosis labels, for example, [Learning Need]. Some diagnoses can be combined for convenience, indicating that two factors may be involved, such as Fluid volume [altered, fluctuation]. It is anticipated that the nurse will choose "what fits." Nurses can be creative as they work with the standardized format, redefining and sharing interventions as they are used with individual patients. Nursing diagnoses should be chosen to meet individual patient needs and should be appropriate for the nurse's practice setting.

Table 2–1
NURSING DIAGNOSES (THROUGH THE EIGHTH NANDA CONFERENCE)

Activity intolerance
Activity intolerance, potential
Adjustment impaired
Airway clearance, ineffective
Anxiety [specific level]*
Aspiration, potential

Body image disturbance
Body temperature, altered, potential
Breastfeeding: ineffective
Breathing pattern, ineffective

Cardiac output, decreased
Communication, impaired verbal
Constipation
Constipation, colonic
Constipation, perceived
Coping, defensive
Coping, individual, ineffective

Decisional conflict (specify)
Denial, ineffective
Diarrhea
Disuse syndrome, potential for
Diversional activity deficit
Dysreflexia

Family coping, compromised, ineffective
Family coping, disabling, ineffective
Family coping, potential for growth
Family processes, altered
Fatigue
Fear
Fluid volume deficit (1) [Regulatory Failure]*
Fluid volume deficit (2) [Active Loss]*
Fluid volume deficit, potential
Fluid volume excess

Gas exchange, impaired
Grieving, anticipatory
Grieving, dysfunctional
Growth and development, altered

Health maintenance, altered
Health-seeking behaviors (specify)
Home maintenance management, impaired
Hopelessness
Hyperthermia
Hypothermia

Incontinence: bowel
Incontinence: functional
Incontinence: reflex
Incontinence: stress
Incontinence: total
Incontinence: urge
Infection, potential for
Injury, potential for

Knowledge deficit [Learning need]* (specify)

Mobility, impaired physical

Noncompliance, specify [Compliance, altered, specify]*
Nutrition, altered, less than body requirements
Nutrition, altered, more than body requirements
Nutrition, potential for more than body requirements

Oral mucous membrane, altered

Pain
Pain, chronic
Parental role conflict
Parenting, altered

(*continued*)

Table 2–1

NURSING DIAGNOSES (THROUGH THE EIGHTH NANDA CONFERENCE) *CONTINUED*

Parenting, altered, potential
Personal identity disturbance
Poisoning, potential for
Post-trauma response
Powerlessness

Rape-trauma syndrome
Rape-trauma syndrome: compound reaction
Rape-trauma syndrome: silent reaction
Role performance, altered

Self-care deficit: feeding, bathing/hygiene, dressing/grooming, toileting
Self-esteem, chronic low
Self-esteem disturbance
Self-esteem, situational low
Sensory-perceptual alterations (specify): visual, auditory, kinesthetic, gustatory, tactile, olfactory
Sexual dysfunction
Sexuality patterns, altered
Skin integrity, impaired
Skin integrity, impaired: potential
Sleep pattern disturbance
Social interaction, impaired
Social isolation
Spiritual distress (distress of the human spirit)
Suffocation, potential for
Swallowing impaired

Thermoregulation, ineffective
Thought processes, altered
Tissue integrity, impaired
Tissue perfusion, altered (specify: cerebral, cardiopulmonary, renal, gastrointestinal, peripheral)
Trauma, potential for

Unilateral neglect

Urinary elimination, altered
Urinary retention [acute/chronic]*

Violence, potential for: directed at self/others

Taxonomy 1 Revised 1989

---

*Information that appears in brackets has been added by the authors to clarify and enhance the use of nursing diagnoses.

CHAPTER 3 DATA COLLECTION

The use of care plans is an accepted way to document patient care. While the content may vary (i.e., nursing input only versus interdisciplinary input, which is a culmination of contributions by many disciplines), most care plans are based on the five steps of the nursing process, which will be discussed at length.

PATIENT ASSESSMENT DATA BASE

Patient assessment is the foundation upon which identification of individual needs, responses, and problems is based. The patient assessment data base is derived from the history-taking interview, the physical examination, and diagnostic studies. Although the philosophy and policies of the health-care agency may affect this process, the data base may be used by numerous/all members of the health-care team.

Interviewing

Interviewing provides a specific set of data (history) that the nurse obtains from the patient and significant others through both conversation (subjective) and observation (objective). The information may be collected during one or more contact periods and should yield, verify, and clarify information. Needed information includes all data (positive and negative) that are relevant to the situation. All participants in the conversation need to know that the information will be used in formulating the plan of patient care. Organization of this data assists in identifying patient problems and desired patient outcomes.

The verbal interchange phase of assessment requires specific interviewing skills. The environment should be quiet, private, and free from distraction. These factors determine the quality of the interview. Techniques, including open-ended and hypothetical questions, reflection, focusing, giving broad openings, offering general leads, exploring, verbalizing the implied, and encouraging evaluation, can help elicit the desired information from patient and/or family. Closed-ended questions (such as Why?), leading, probing, and agreeing/disagreeing usually are not helpful in eliciting information. These types of questions will be reviewed so the nurse understands and can avoid them.

An open-ended question, such as "How do you feel about your new medication?," might elicit valuable information, such as "I don't want to take it." "Explain the injection techniques to me" may lead to "I clean it with soap, alcohol, pinch the skin, and inject the medicine." These questions allow the person maximal freedom in responding by imposing no limitations on how the question may be answered and can produce considerable information.

Conversely, the closed-ended question, such as "Do you take your medicine?" (patient responds "No") or "How long have you been taking insulin?" (patient responds "3 years"), allows the person little or no freedom in choosing a response. Typically, there are only one or two possible answers to the question. The interviewer remains in close control over the interview because of the rigid structure. The closed-ended question is helpful in an emergency when it is necessary to gather information in a short time. If time remains at the end of the interview, it is important to ask the patient to explain the answers to these questions in greater detail. Often, patients feel frustrated or manipulated in an interview dominated by the closed-ended question that fails to give them an opportunity to explain.

Clarifying, focusing, and reflecting, on the other hand, provide an opportunity for the interviewee to explain more fully what the meaning of the answer is for better understanding. These responses move language from the abstract to the concrete by requiring specific and descriptive terms in the patient's answer.

The hypothetical question helps the nurse learn how the patient might handle a particular situation. These include "What would you do if you felt dizzy?" and "What would you do if you noticed a rash on your body?" These questions may be very useful in determining the extent to which the patient has learned previously presented material.

Reflecting or "mirroring" responses are useful in getting at underlying meanings that might not be verbalized clearly. As an example, the patient may say, "Some days I'd like to throw this needle out the window." A mirror response might be, "You feel angry about the needle?" Now the patient is encouraged to verbalize what s/he is actually angry about. This response is nonevaluative and nonthreatening.

Leading questions typically suggest the desired response, such as "The infection seems to be getting better, don't you agree?" and reduce the range of responses, as the interviewee most commonly agrees with any leading statement. Highly emotional terms (e.g., "Where did you learn that injection technique?") also suggest the desired response, are heard as challenging, and may provoke the interviewee to "attack" or become defensive.

At the conclusion of the interview, the nurse summarizes the data to be sure the patient, family, and nurse have the same understanding of the information.

The nurse-interviewer needs to listen attentively to what the patient and family are saying. It is also important to separate the talker from the topic. If the interviewee is dressed in shabby clothes or talks in a monotone, the nurse must react not to the person but to the message. The nurse also listens for whole thoughts and ideas, not merely for isolated facts. Facts themselves are not as important as the ideas that bind them together. For example, a diabetic patient may tell the nurse facts about his/her diet and daily insulin injections, but the whole thought includes the idea that the patient does not accept his/her diabetes and is really not following his/her diet closely. Also, the nurse can use silence and acceptance, saving comments until the speaker is completely finished. If the nurse-interviewer begins to react emotionally, the rest of the patient's message is usually lost to the nurse. The nurse needs to react empathetically and nonjudgmentally to information from the patient.

Physical Examination

During this aspect of information gathering, the nurse exercises perceptual and observational skills using the senses of sight, hearing, touch, and smell. Sight and hearing are used to elicit many responses in doing a head-to-toe examination. Touch can elicit data about muscle tension, moisture, and body temperature. Smell can also elicit data about various body odors that may be significant in diagnosis or initiating certain nursing actions. Physical examination skills vary from basic to advanced; however, the nurse needs to know the normal physical and emotional characteristics well enough to be able to recognize deviations. The duration and depth of any physical examination depend on circumstances such as the condition of the patient and urgency of the situation. Several different formats are available. Data can be collected according to body systems being examined (medical model) or by a nursing model, (e.g., Diagnostic Divisions (Table 3–1), Functional Health Patterns). Findings may be recorded according to subjective data (i.e., reports) and objective data (e.g., exhibits) or activity involved (i.e., inspection, palpation, etc.).

Diagnostic Studies

Laboratory studies are included as part of the information gathering process. Some tests are used to diagnose disease, while others are useful in following the course of a disease or in adjusting therapies. In some cases, the relationship of the test to the pathologic physiology is unclear as a result of the interrelationships among the various organs and systems of the body. Test results should be integrated with the history and physical findings, and the nurse needs to be aware of significant findings to report to the physician, and/or to initiate specific nursing actions, for example, holding medication and notifying the physician of an elevated serum drug level.

In this book, we have chosen to use a nursing framework Diagnostic Divisions as seen in Table 3–2 A, B, and C to achieve a nursing focus. These divisions (reflecting a blending of Maslow's Hierarchy of Needs and a self-care philosophy) serve as the outline for data collection, which directs the nurse to the appropriate corresponding nursing diagnoses. Because these divisions are based on human responses/needs and not specific "systems," information may occasionally be recorded in more than one area. For this reason, the nurse is encouraged to pursue all avenues/leads and collect as much data as possible before choosing the nursing diagnosis that best reflects the patient's situation. The results (synthesis) of the collected data are written in succinct, descriptive paragraphs, or concise diagnostic statements in construction of the patient care plan.

Table 3–1
DIAGNOSTIC DIVISIONS

After data have been collected, and areas of concern/need have been identified, the nurse is directed to the Diagnostic Divisions to review the list of nursing diagnoses that fall within the individual categories. This will assist the nurse in choosing the specific diagnostic label to describe the data accurately. Then with the addition of etiology (when known) and signs and symptoms, the patient problem statement emerges.

Activity/Rest

Activity intolerance, potential
Activity intolerance, potential for
Disuse syndrome, potential for
Diversional activity deficit
Fatigue
Sleep pattern disturbance

Circulation

Cardiac output, decreased
Dysreflexia
Tissue perfusion, altered: (specify) (renal, cerebral, cardiopulmonary, gastrointestinal, peripheral)

Ego Integrity

Adjustment, impaired
Anxiety (specify level)
Body image disturbance
Coping, defensive
Coping, ineffective individual
Decisional conflict (specify)
Denial, ineffective
Fear
Grieving, anticipatory
Grieving, dysfunctional
Hopelessness
Personal identity disturbance
Post-trauma response
Powerlessness
Rape-trauma syndrome
Rape-trauma syndrome: compound reaction
Rape-trauma syndrome: silent reaction
Self-esteem disturbance

Self-esteem, chronic low
Self-esteem, situational low
Spiritual distress (distress of the human spirit)

Elimination

Bowel incontinence
Constipation
Constipation, colonic
Constipation, perceived
Diarrhea
Incontinence, functional
Incontinence, reflex
Incontinence, stress
Incontinence, total
Incontinence, urge
Urinary elimination, altered patterns
Urinary retention [acute/chronic]*

Food/Fluid

Breastfeeding, ineffective
Fluid volume deficit, (1) [regulatory failure]*
Fluid volume deficit, (2) [active loss]*
Fluid volume deficit, potential
Fluid volume excess
Nutrition, altered: less than body requirements
Nutrition, altered: more than body requirements
Nutrition, altered: potential for more than body requirements
Oral mucous membranes, altered
Swallowing, impaired

Hygiene

Self-care deficit: feeding, bathing/hygiene, dressing/grooming, toileting

Neurosensory

Sensory-perceptual alterations (specify) (visual, auditory, kinesthetic, gustatory, tactile, olfactory)
Thought processes, altered
Unilateral neglect

(*continued*)

Table 3–1
DIAGNOSTIC DIVISIONS—*CONTINUED*

Pain/Comfort

Pain
Pain, chronic

Respiration

Airway clearance, ineffective
Aspiration, potential for
Breathing pattern, ineffective
Gas exchange, impaired

Safety

Body temperature, altered, potential
Health maintenance, altered
Home maintenance management, impaired
Hyperthermia
Hypothermia
Infection, potential for
Injury, potential for
Mobility, impaired physical
Poisoning, potential for
Skin integrity, impaired
Skin integrity, impaired, potential
Suffocation, potential for
Thermoregulation, ineffective
Tissue integrity, impaired
Trauma, potential for
Violence, potential for: self-directed or directed at others

Sexuality (Component of Social Interaction)

Sexual dysfunction
Sexuality patterns, altered

Social Interaction

Communication, impaired verbal
Coping, family: potential for growth
Coping, ineffective family: compromised
Coping, ineffective family: disabling
Family processes, altered
Parental role conflict
Parenting, altered
Parenting, altered, potential

Role performance, altered
Social interaction, impaired
Social isolation

Teaching/Learning

Growth and development, altered
Health seeking behaviors (specify)
Knowledge deficit [learning need]* (specify)
Noncompliance [compliance, altered]* (specify)

---

*Information that appears in brackets has been added by the authors to clarify and enhance the use of nursing diagnoses.

Table 3–2A
ADULT MEDICAL/SURGICAL ASSESSMENT TOOL

This is a suggested guide/tool for development by an individual/institution to create a data base reflecting Diagnostic Divisions of Nursing Diagnoses. Although the divisions are alphabetized for ease of presentation, they can be prioritized or rearranged to meet individual needs.

Name: ______________________

Age: ____________ DOB: ____________

Sex: ____________ Race: ____________

Admission date: ______ Time: ______ From: ______

Source of information: ______ Reliability (1–4): ______

Family member/significant other: ____________

ACTIVITY/REST

Subjective

Occupation: ______ Usual activities/hobbies: ______

Leisure-time activities: ____________

Complaints of boredom: ____________

Limitations imposed by condition: ____________

Sleep: Hours: ______ Naps: ______ Aids: ______

Insomnia: ________ Related to: ________

Rested upon awakening: ____________

Objective

Observed response to activity: Cardiovascular: ______

Respiratory: ______

Mental status (e.g., withdrawn/lethargic): ________

Neuromuscular assessment:

Muscle mass/tone: ____________

Posture: ________ Tremors: ________

ROM: ________ Strength: ________

Deformity: ________ Other: ________

CIRCULATION

Subjective

History of: Hypertension: ______ Heart trouble: ______
Rheumatic fever: ___ Ankle/leg edema: ___
Phlebitis: __________ Slow healing: ______
Claudication: ______ Other: ____________

Extremities: Numbness: ________ Tingling: __________

Cough/hemoptysis: ________________________________

Change in frequency/amount of urine: _______________

Objective

B/P: R: Lying: ________ Sit: ________ Stand: ________
L: Lying: ________ Sit: ________ Stand: ________
Pulse pressure: _______ Auscultatory gap: _______

Pulse (palpation): Carotid: ________ Temporal: ________
Jugular: _______________ Radial: __________________
Femoral: _______________ Popliteal: _______________
Post tibial: ____________ Dorsalis pedis: ___________

Cardiac (palpation): PMI: __________________________
Thrill: _________________ Heaves: _________________

Heart sounds: Rate: _____ Rhythm: _____ Quality: _____
Friction rub: ______________ Murmur: _____________

Breath sounds: ____________________________________

Vascular bruit: (specify) ____________________________

Jugular vein distention: ____________________________

Extremities: Temperature: _________ Color: _________
Capillary refill: _________________________________
Homan's sign: ____________ Varicosities: ___________
Nails (describe abnormalities): ______________________
Distribution/quality of hair: _______________________

Color/cyanosis: Overall: ____ Mucous membranes: ____

(*continued*)

Table 3–2A

ADULT MEDICAL/SURGICAL ASSESSMENT TOOL—*CONTINUED*

Lips: ______

Nail beds: ______ Conjunctiva: ______ Sclera: ______

Diaphoresis: ______

EGO INTEGRITY

Subjective

Report of stress factors: ______

Ways of handling stress: ______

Financial concerns: ______

Relationship status: ______

Cultural factors: ______

Religion: ______ Practicing: ______

Lifestyle: ______ Recent changes: ______

Feelings of: helplessness: ______ hopelessness: ______

powerlessness: ______

Objective

Emotional status (check those that apply):

Calm: ______ Anxious: ______

Angry: ______ Withdrawn: ______

Fearful: ______ Irritable: ______

Restive: ______ Euphoric: ______

Other (specify): ______

Observed physiologic responses(s): ______

ELIMINATION

Subjective

Usual bowel pattern: ______ Laxative use: ______

Character of stool: ______ Last BM: ______________

History of bleeding: ____ Hemorrhoids: ___________

Constipation: __________ Diarrhea: ______________

Usual voiding pattern: ___ Incontinence: ___ When: ___

Urgency: _____ Frequency: _____ Retention: _____

Character of urine: ______________________________

Pain/burning/difficulty voiding: ___________________

History of kidney/bladder disease: _________________

Objective

Abdomen tender: ________ Soft/firm: ______________

Palpable mass: ________ Size/girth: ______________

Bowel sounds: ___________________________________

Hemorrhoids (per rectal exam):

Internal: _____________ External: ______________

Bladder palpable: ________ Overflow voiding: ________

FOOD/FLUID

Subjective

Usual diet (type): ________ # meals daily: ___________

Last meal/intake: ________ Dietary pattern: _________

Loss of appetite: ________ Nausea/vomiting: _________

Heartburn/indigestion: ________ Related to: _________

Relieved by: ___________________________________

Allergy/food intolerance: __________________________

Mastication/swallowing problems: __________________

Dentures: upper: ____________ lower: ____________

Usual weight: _________ Changes in weight: _________

Use of diuretics: ________________________________

Objective

Current weight: _____________ Height: _____________

(*continued*)

Table 3–2A
ADULT MEDICAL/SURGICAL ASSESSMENT TOOL—*CONTINUED*

Body build: ______________ Skin turgor: ______________

Mucous membranes moist/dry: ______________

Hernia/masses: ______________

Edema: General: ______________ Dependent: ______________

Periorbital: ______________ Ascites: ______________

Jugular vein distention: ______________

Thyroid enlarged: ______________ Halitosis: ______________

Condition of teeth/gums: ______________

Appearance of tongue: ______________

Mucous membranes: ______________

Bowel sounds (previously assessed): ______________

Breath sounds (previously assessed): ______________

Urine S/A or Chemstix: ______________

HYGIENE

Subjective

Activities of daily living: Independent: ______________

Dependent (specify):

Mobility: ______________ Feeding: ______________

Hygiene: ______________ Dressing: ______________

Toileting: ______________ Other: ______________

Equipment/prosthetic devices required: ______________

Assistance provided by: ______________

Preferred time of bath: __________ AM __________ PM

Objective

General appearance: ______________

Manner of dress: ________ **Personal habits:** ________

Body odor: ________ **Condition of scalp:** ________

Presence of vermin: ________________

NEUROSENSORY

Subjective

Fainting spells/dizziness: ________________

Headaches: Location: ________ **Frequency:** ________

Tingling/numbness/weakness (location): ________

Stroke (residual effects): ________________

Seizures: ______ **Aura:** ______ **How controlled:** ______

Eyes: Vision loss: R ________ **L** ________

Glaucoma: ________ **Cataract:** ________

Ears: Hearing loss: R ________ **L** ________

Nose: Epistaxis: ________ **Sense of smell:** ________

Objective

Mental status:

Oriented/disoriented: Time: ________________

Place: ________ **Person:** ________

Alert: ________ **Drowsy:** ________

Lethargic: ________ **Stuporous:** ________

Comatose: ________ **Other:** ________

Cooperative: ________ **Combative:** ________

Delusions: ________ **Hallucinations:** ________

Affect (describe): ________________

Memory: Recent: ________ **Remote:** ________

Speech pattern: ________ **Content:** ________

(*continued*)

Table 3–2A
ADULT MEDICAL/SURGICAL ASSESSMENT TOOL—*CONTINUED*

Word choice: __________ Congruence: __________

Glasses: ______ Contacts: ______ Hearing aids: ______

Pupil size/reaction: R ______________ L ______________

Facial droop: ______________ Swallowing: ______________

Handgrip/release: R ______________ L ______________

Posturing: ______________________________________

Deep tendon reflexes: __________ Paralysis: __________

PAIN/COMFORT

Subjective

Location: ______________ Intensity (1–10): ________

Frequency: ______________ Quality: ______________

Duration: ______________ Radiation: ______________

Precipitating factors: ______________________________

How relieved: ____________________________________

Objective

Facial grimacing: ________ Guarding affected area: ___

Emotional response: ______ Narrowed focus: ________

RESPIRATION

Subjective

Dyspnea (related to): ______________________________

Cough/sputum: ____________________________________

History of Bronchitis: ____ Asthma: ______________

Tuberculosis: __________ Emphysema: ____________

Recurrent pneumonia: __________ Other: __________

Exposure to noxious fumes: ______________________

Smoker: _______ **Pk/day:** _______ **# of years:** _______

Use of respiratory aids: _________ **Oxygen:** _________

Objective

Respiratory: Rate: ______________________________

Depth: _______________ **Symmetry:** _______________

Use of accessory muscles: ______ **Nasal flaring:** ______

Fremitis: ______________________________________

Breath sounds: _________________________________

Egophony: ______________________________________

Cyanosis: __________ **Clubbing of fingers:** __________

Sputum characteristics: ___________________________

Mentation/restlessness: ___________________________

Other: ____

SAFETY

Subjective

Allergies/sensitivity: __________ **Reaction:** __________

Previous alteration of immune system: ____________

Cause: _______________________________________

History of sexually transmitted disease (date/type): ____

Blood transfusion # ____________ **When:** ____________

Reaction (describe): ______________________________

History of accidental injuries: _______________________

Fractures/dislocations: ____________________________

Arthritis/unstable joints: __________________________

Back problems: ___________________________________

Changes in moles: _______ **Enlarged nodes:** _________

Impaired: Vision: _______ **Hearing:** _______________

Prosthesis: _________ **Ambulatory devices:** _________

Expressions of ideation of violence (self/others): _______

(*continued*)

Table 3–2A
ADULT MEDICAL/SURGICAL ASSESSMENT TOOL—*CONTINUED*

Objective

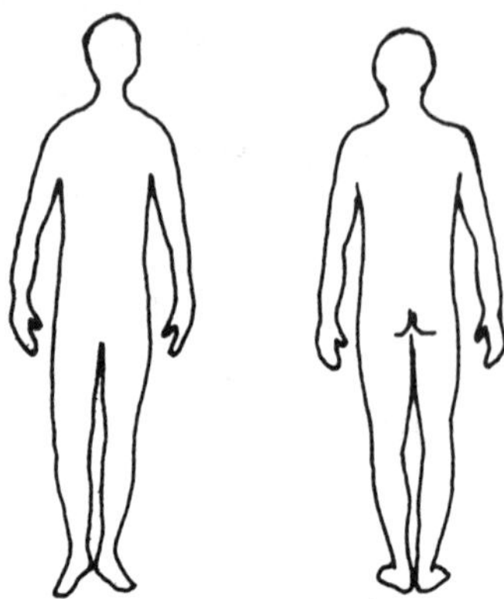

Temperature: ______________ **Diaphoresis:** ______________

Skin integrity: ____

Scars: ________________ **Rashes:** ________________

Lacerations: ____________ **Ulcerations:** ____________

Ecchymosis: ____________ **Blisters:** ______________

Burns, degree/percent: ______________________________

General strength: ____________ **Muscle tone:** __________

Gait: __________________ **ROM:** __________________

Paresthesia/paralysis: ______________________________

SEXUALITY

Sexual concerns: ____________________________________

Female

Subjective

Age at menarche: __________ **Length of cycle:** __________

Duration: __________ **Last menstrual period:** __________

Menopause: __________ Vaginal discharge: __________

Bleeding between periods: __________________________

Practices breast self-exam: _____ Last PAP smear: _____

Method of birth control: ____________________________

Objective

Breast exam: ______________________________________

Vaginal warts/lesions: ______________________________

Male

Subjective

Penile discharge: ________ Prostate disorder: ________

Vasectomy: _____________ Use of condoms: _________

Practice self-exam: Breast: ________ Testicles: ________

Last proctoscopic exam: _____ Last prostate exam: _____

Objective

Exam: Breast: _____________ Testicles: _____________

SOCIAL INTERACTIONS

Subjective

Marital status: ________ Years in relationship: ________

Living with: ______________________________________

Concerns/stresses: ______________________________

Extended family: __________________________________

Other support person(s): ___________________________

Role within family structure: ________________________

Report of problems related to illness/condition: ________

Coping behaviors: ________________________________

Do others depend on you for assistance?: _____________

How are they managing?: _________________________

(continued)

Table 3–2A

ADULT MEDICAL/SURGICAL ASSESSMENT TOOL—*CONTINUED*

Frequency of social contacts (other than work): ________

Objective

Speech: Clear: ______________ Slurred: ______________

Unintelligible: ______________ Aphasic: ______________

Unusual speech pattern/impairment: ______________

Laryngectomy: ____________ Speech aids: ____________

Verbal/nonverbal communication with family/S.O.(s):

____

Family interaction (behavioral) pattern: ______________

TEACHING/LEARNING

Subjective

Dominant language (specify): ________ Literate: ________

Education level: ____________________________

Learning disabilities (specify): ______________________

Cognitive limitations (specify): ______________________

Health beliefs/practices: ____________________________

Special health-care practices: _______________________

Familial risk factors (indicate relationship):

Diabetes: ______________ Tuberculosis: ______________

Heart disease: __________ Stroke: ______________

High BP: ______________ Epilepsy: ______________

Kidney disease: _________ Cancer: ______________

Mental illness: _________ Other (specify): ___________

Prescribed medications: (circle last dose)

Drug:	Dose:	Times:
___________	___________	___________
___________	___________	___________

Take regularly: ____________ Purpose: ____________

____________ ____________

____________ ____________

Non-prescription drugs: OTC: ____________

Street drugs: ________ Smokeless tobacco: ________

Use of alcohol (amount/frequency): ____________

Admitting diagnosis (physician): ____________

Reason for hospitalization (patient): ____________

History of current complaint: ____________

Patient expectations of this hospitalization: ____________

Previous illnesses and/or hospitalizations/surgeries:

____

Evidence of failure to improve: ____________

Last complete physical exam: ________ By: ________

DISCHARGE PLAN CONSIDERATIONS

Date data obtained: ____________

1. Anticipated date of discharge: ____________
2. Resources available: Persons: ____________

   Financial: ____________
3. Do you anticipate changes in your living situation after discharge?: ____________
4. If Yes: Areas that may require alteration/ assistance:

   Food preparation: ________ Shopping: ________

   Transportation: ________ Ambulation: ________

   Medication/IV therapy: ___ Treatments: ________

   Wound care: ________ Supplies: ________

   Self-care assistance (specify): ____________

   Physical layout of home (specify): ____________

   Homemaker assistance (specify): ____________

   Living facility other than home (specify): ________

Sections of the basic nursing history may be altered/expanded to meet the needs of any patient population, for example, psychiatric or obstetric as in Tables 3–2B and 3–2C.

Table 3–2B

EXCERPTS FROM PSYCHIATRIC ASSESSMENT TOOL

EGO INTEGRITY

Subjective

What kind of person are you?: (positive/negative, etc.): _______________

What do you think of your body?: _______________

How would you rate your self-esteem (1–10)?: _______________

What are your moods?: depressed: _______________

guilty: _______________ **unreal:** _______________

ups/downs: _______________ **apathetic:** _______________

separated from world: _______________ **detached:** _______________

Are you a nervous person?: _______________

Are your feelings easily hurt?: _______________

Report of stress factors: _______________

Previous patterns of coping with stress: _______________

Financial concerns: _______________

Relationship status: _______________

Cultural factors: _______________

Lifestyle: _______________

Significant losses/changes (date): _______________

Stage of grief/manifestations of loss: _______________

Religion: _______________ **Practicing:** _______________

Objective

Emotional status (check those that apply):

Calm: _______________ **Friendly:** _______________

Cooperative: ________ Evasive: ________

Fearful: ________ Anxious: ________

Irritable: ________ Withdrawn: ________

Restive: ________ Passive: ________

Dependent: ________ Euphoric: ________

Angry/hostile: ________ Other (specify): ________

Consistency of behavior: ________

Verbal: ________

Nonverbal: ________

Characteristics of speech: ________

Motor behaviors: ________ Posturing: ________

Under/overactive: ________ Stereotypic: ________

Defense mechanisms:

Projection: ________ Denial: ________

Undoing: ________ Rationalization: ________

Passive aggressive: ________ Repression: ________

Intellectualization: ________ Somatization: ________

Regression: ________ Identification: ________

Introjection: ________ Reaction formation: ________

Isolation: ________ Displacement: ________

Substitution: ________ Sublimation: ________

Observed physiologic response(s): ________

Other: ________

NEUROSENSORY

Subjective

Dreamlike states: ________ Walking in sleep: ________

Automatic writing: ________

Believe/feel you are another person: ________

Reports perception different than others: ________

(*continued*)

Table 3–2B
EXCERPTS FROM PSYCHIATRIC ASSESSMENT TOOL—*CONTINUED*

Objective

Mental status: ______

Memory: Immediate: ______

Recent: ______ **Remote:** ______

Intellectual function: ______

Judgment: ______

Comprehension: ______

Thought processes (Assessed through speech): ______

Patterns of speech: ______

Content: ______

Delusions: ______ **Hallucinations:** ______

Illusions: ______

Rate or flow: ______

Clear, logical progression: ______

Expression: ______

Speech: Clear: ______ **Slurred:** ______

Unintelligible: ______ **Aphasic:** ______

Unusual speech pattern/impairment: ______

Mood: ______

Affect: ______ **Appropriateness:** ______

Intensity: ______ **Range:** ______

Insight: ______

Table 3–2C
EXCERPTS FROM OBSTETRICAL ASSESSMENT TOOL

Prenatal Assessment

SAFETY

Subjective

German measles: ______

Exposure to radiation: ______

Previous obstetrical problems:

PIH: ______ Kidney: ______

Hemorrhage: ______ Cardiac: ______

Diabetes: ______ Other: ______

ABO/Rh sensitivity: ______

Objective

Fetal: Heart rate: ______ Location: ______

Method of auscultation: ______

Fundal height: ______ Estimated gestation: ______

Movement: ______ Ballottement: ______

Blood type/Rh: Maternal: ______ Paternal: ______

Screens: Sickle cell: ______ Rubella: ______

Hepatitis: ______ AFP: ______

Serology syphilis: Pos ______ Neg ______

Cervical/rectal culture: Pos ______ Neg ______

Vaginal warts/lesions: ______

SEXUALITY

Subjective

OB history: Gravida: ______

Para: ______ Abortions: ______

Now living: ______ Full term: ______

(*continued*)

Table 3–2C

EXCERPTS FROM OBSTETRIC ASSESSMENT TOOL—*CONTINUED*

Premature: ________ Multiple births: ________

Preg #	Year	Place of Del	Length Gestation	Length Labor
____	____	____	______	____
____	____	____	______	____

Type Deliv.	Born A/D	Wt	Complications Mat/Fetal
____	____	____	________
____	____	____	________

Objective

Pelvic: Vulva: ________ Perineum: ________

Vagina: ________ Cervix: ________

Uterus: ________ Adnexal: ________

Diagonal conjugate: ______________ cm

Transverse diameter: Outlet: __________ cm

Shape of sacrum: ________ Arch: ________

Coccyx: ________ SS notch: ________

Ischial spines: ______________

	Adequate	Borderline	Contracted
Inlet	____	____	____
Mid	____	____	____
Outlet	____	____	____

Prognosis for Delivery: ______________

Breast exam: ________ Nipples: ________

Serology test: ______________

Intrapartal Assessment — The intrapartal admission assessment would consider the following:

PAIN/COMFORT

Subjective

Onset of regular uterine contractions (date/time): ______

Location of contractile pain:

Front: ______________ Sacral area: ______________

Degree of discomfort: Mild: ______________________

Moderate: ______________ Severe: ______________

How relieved: Breathing/relaxation techniques: _______

Positioning: ____________ Sacral rubs: ____________

Effleurage: ______________________________________

SAFETY

Subjective

Health status of living children: _____________________

Month of first prenatal visit: _______________________

Previous/current obstetric problems/treatment:

PIH: ________________ Kidney: ________________

Hemorrhage: __________ Cardiac: _______________

Diabetes: ____________ Infection (specify): _______

Uterine surgery: _______ UTI: __________________

ABO/Rh Sensitivity: ____________________________

Anemia: ___________________________________

Length of time since last pregnancy: ________________

Type of previous delivery: ________________________

Objective

Fetal status: Heart rate: __________________________

Location: _____________________________________

Method of auscultation: ________________________

(continued)

Table 3–2C

EXCERTS FROM OBSTETRICAL ASSESSMENT TOOL—*CONTINUED*

Fundal height: _______ Estimated gestation: _______

Activity/movement: ____________________

Fetal assessment testing (Y/N): _______________

Date/test: _____________ Results: ____________

Labor status: Cervical dilation: _______________

Effacement: ____________________________

Fetal: Descent: __________ Engagement: __________

Presentation: ______________ Lie: ______________

Position: ___________________________________

Fetal: Descent: __________ Engagement: __________

Presentation: ______________ Lie: ______________

Position: ___________________________________

Membranes: Intact: _____ Ruptured date/time: _____

Nitrazine test: ______ Amount of drainage: ______

Character: Clear: __________ Cloudy: __________

Meconium stained: _________________________

CHAPTER 4

CARE PLAN CONSTRUCTION

Once the patient data have been gathered, it is the responsibility of the registered nurse to initiate/develop a plan of care based on the individual needs and concerns of the specific patient. Care plans are not "busy work" but can actually save valuable nursing time as the goals of care and interventions to achieve these individual goals are identified to promote optimal patient recovery in a timely manner. This plan of care needs to be written to:

- *provide continuity* of care from nurse to nurse, shift to shift, or even one unit/care setting to another;
- *enhance communication* because written plan is a permanent part of the record and provides the same information for each individual who reads it;
- *assist with setting priorities* for the shift work schedule;
- *support documentation of the nursing process* by providing reminders of what needs to be charted and when evaluations should be done; and
- *serve as a teaching tool* that shares nurses' expertise and fosters professional growth as nurses learn what interventions are successful.

PROBLEM/IDENTIFICATION FOCUS (NURSING DIAGNOSIS)

Accurate diagnosis of a patient problem can provide a standard for nursing action, understood by all who use the plan of care, thus improving coordination and delivery of care. Nursing diagnosis can provide a uniform way of identifying, focusing on, and labeling specific phenomena to deal with individual problems/responses.

A nursing diagnosis may be a physical, sociologic, or psychologic finding. Physical nursing diagnoses include those that pertain to circulation, ventilation, elimination, and so forth. Psychosocial nursing diagnoses include those that pertain to the mind, emotion, or lifestyle/relationships.

The steps involved in the process of problem/focus identification and choosing nursing diagnosis are:

1. Collection of a data base.
2. Analyzing and reviewing the data for relevant information (positive findings/abnormalities), for conflicts (differences in data that normally reinforce each other), or for negative findings/information expected to exist that does not (e.g., complaints of pain in the right upper quadrant, but does not flinch/guard on abdominal palpation).
3. Synthesizing (combining/organizing) the data to provide a comprehensive picture of the patient into nursing diagnostic problems/concerns, focus.
4. Comparing and contrasting the relationships among the diagnoses according to established criteria (e.g., etiology, risk factors, defining characteristics). This step is crucial to the creation of individual patient problem statements/focus as the nurse determines relation-

ships and identifies the causative factors within or between categories.

5. Based on the data obtained, the nursing diagnosis is combined with the etiology and signs/symptoms to create the *patient problem statement/focus* (e.g., pain related to inflammatory process as evidenced by muscle guarding, restlessness, narrowed focus, grimacing).

Once possible/probable nursing diagnoses are identified, they are listed according to priority and classified according to status, such as, active, inactive, or resolved. Active diagnoses are those that require some form of current action or intervention. Inactive/potential diagnoses are those that may occur/recur. Resolved diagnoses are those that no longer need action.

PATIENT OUTCOMES/ EVALUATION CRITERIA

Once a patient problem has been identified, the goals for treatment/discharge criteria are established and are broadly stated reflecting the general outcome towards which the patient is expected to progress. The next step in the treatment plan is the formation of specific expected measurable outcomes, which are defined as responses that may be achievable, are desired by the patient, and can be attained within a defined time period given the present situation and resources. Therefore, useful patient outcome statements need to:

1. Be specific.
2. Be realistic.
3. Consider the patient's circumstances and desires.
4. Indicate a time frame.
5. Provide measurable evaluation criteria for de-

termination of success or failure in achieving the desired outcome.

Desired outcomes are written by listing items/behaviors to observe which can determine that a positive/acceptable outcome has been achieved (e.g., Verbalizes understanding of disease process and potential complications). This serves as the evaluation tool. Action verbs are used when the patient or nurse is asked to perform an action (e.g., Ambulates with use of cane). Some examples of measurable verbs are: discusses, states, identifies, administers, explains, reports. Time elements also provide measurable criteria (e.g., Ambulates with cane without assistance within three days).

When outcomes are properly written, they provide direction for planning and validating the choice of interventions (e.g., Identifies individual nutritional needs and formulates dietary plan based on these needs within 48 hours). From this outcome, the nurse knows that the patient's level of knowledge needs to be assessed, individual needs identified, and information presented to provide the patient with the tools necessary to formulate a dietary plan. A goal of improving self-esteem may call for desired measurable outcomes ranging from weight loss to increased verbalization of self-worth. If the expected measurable outcomes do not seem to relate logically to the goals for treatment/discharge, it should be questioned whether they are a valid component of the treatment plan.

Outcomes involve different time frames, that is: long-term, intermediate, or short-term. Long-term outcomes indicate the overall direction for actions as a result of the interventions of the health-care team and/or patient. These outcomes may not be achieved before discharge. Intermediate outcomes are shorter range activities directed toward accomplishing the long-range goal(s). Short-term outcomes are more specific guides for action in the use of the nursing process and usually must be met before discharge or movement to a less acute level of care, supervision, or support. Depending on the patient's anticipated length of stay/care, a short-term goal may be evaluated within a few hours or several therapeutic sessions, which could reflect several calendar weeks. If the goal is to be met within the originating shift, it need not be written on the care plan but would be indicated in the progress note. If the goal is not accomplished by the end of the shift, it then would be added to the care plan with a new time frame so that oncoming nurses can continue to work toward the outcome.

All desired measurable outcomes should tell the reader specifically what the patient is working on or doing. With this in mind, there is a simple and straightforward method of determining if the expected measurable outcome is correctly written: The nurse should ask his/herself if the patient can be observed in the performance of the behavior indicated. If the answer is no, the desired measurable outcome should be modified. Below are several examples of desired measurable outcomes, with notation:

1. "The patient understands treatment needs within 48 hours."
   Note: This patient outcome states a clear time line, but can a patient's "understanding" be measured? This outcome needs to be more specific.
2. "The patient correctly performs insulin administration and explains reasons for the actions within 48 hours."
   Note: This is a well-written outcome that is observable, measurable and is time-limited.
3. "The patient requires no reminders from staff regarding dietary restrictions within 3 days."

Note: This outcome tells what the staff will do, not what the patient will do.

4. "The patient lists individual dietary restrictions and makes appropriate choices from daily menu within 3 days."
   Note: This outcome is observable and easy to document.
5. "The patient receives fewer restrictions for defying staff instructions during the next 2 weeks."
   Note: What exactly is the definition of "fewer"? A specific number is better. What constitutes *defiance* and what is the patient *doing*? According to this desired measurable outcome, the patient *receives* fewer restrictions, which places the patient in an essentially passive role. Good measurable outcomes state what the patient actively *does*.
6. "The patient decreases self-abusive acts from the current rate of five incidents per week to no more than two per week within 2 weeks."
   Note: Incidents of self-abuse are major events that are observable, well documented, and easy to track. This outcome is also time-limited and is a well-written desired measurable outcome.

As goals are evaluated, it becomes apparent that they may have been met, partially met, or may have not been met at all. Goals are guides to show the direction of care and not meant to be a guarantee. As progress is made, and goals reviewed, it may become apparent that the patient has changed in a direction that was not anticipated and that a change in treatment is indicated. This is not a failure on the part of the caregivers, but rather a sign that care is being evaluated and changed on an ongoing basis to meet the needs of the patient. As problems change and new problems are identified, goals will be resolved and/or changed.

The patient outcomes are only a part of the overall health-care outcome(s). Each discipline involved in assisting the patient will have individual outcomes that contribute to the overall goal(s). The challenge is to write meaningful outcomes that can be understood and used by all colleagues in health care and that avoid multidisciplinary conflicts. Outcomes may be an indicator of further need for care/supervision, possibly in an alternate setting such as the home, a day care program, clinic, or an extended care facility.

Some agencies separate patient outcomes from nursing goals. Nursing goals may represent outcomes in the patient who has little individual responsibility in achieving them, (e.g., airway clearance in a comatose patient or control of gastric bleeding and improved cardiac output). These goals are more likely to be achieved by intervention of health team members. However, since the well-being of the patient is dependent on the achievement of these nurses/patient goals, they are combined here for simplicity.

NURSING INTERVENTIONS

After the information is gathered, the problems/concerns identified, and the outcomes formulated, actions are selected that can be expected to achieve the desired outcomes. In the patient care plan, this basic unit is known as an intervention or action.

Nursing interventions are prescriptions for specific behaviors expected from the nurses and/or other members of the health team and have the intent of individualizing care. The expectation is that the prescribed behavior/action benefits the patient in a predictable way related to the identified diagnosis and desired outcome. Nursing actions may be independent or collaborative and encompass orders from nursing, medicine, and other disciplines.

Independent nursing actions are an integral part of the care planning process. The educational background/expertise of the nurse, established protocols/standards of care, and areas of practice (rural/urban, acute/community care settings) can influence whether an individual intervention is actually an independent nursing function or one requiring collaboration. Interdependent/collaborative actions are based on the medical regimen as well as on suggestions/orders from other disciplines involved with the care of the patient.

The medical plan of care is incorporated as nurses implement physician orders and reveals the appropriate interventions required in the implementation of the medical plan (e.g., Administer analgesic medications). In addition, nursing interventions show which actions need to be performed to achieve nursing goals related to the medical plan (e.g., Monitor effects of drug/other medical interventions).

Written nursing interventions provide the means for guiding ongoing nursing care. Interventions begin with an action verb, communicating a specific behavior (e.g., instruct, assess, perform). Content area deals with the "what, where, and how" of the intervention, especially when continuity and repetition are described (e.g., time elements may be included indicating "when, how often, or how long" an intervention is to be implemented depending on patient need and/or institutional policy, such as every 2 hours × 4 then qid).

Two examples of appropriately written outcomes followed by examples of interventions are as follows:

1. Patient Outcome/Evaluation Criteria:
   Ms. Jones correctly performs insulin administration and explains reasons for the actions within 4 days.
   Interventions:
   A. Show filmstrip "Managing Your Diabetes."
   B. Review information presented.
   C. Provide step-by-step diagram for "Insulin Self-administration."
   D. Demonstrate process, correlating reasons for each action.
   E. Observe patient in preparing and administering insulin injection for three consecutive mornings.
2. Patient Outcome/Evaluation Criteria:
   Mr. Smith ceases inappropriate behaviors when confronted by the staff at least 50 percent of the time during the next week.
   Interventions:
   A. Confront the patient's rude and vulgar interactions with peers in a supportive manner, discussing current desired measurable outcomes with him.
   B. Document in the progress notes each occasion that the patient is confronted, describing the behavior, what he was doing, and his response to staff intervention.

These interventions clearly state what the nurse/staff is to do and can be easily followed by whoever is caring for the patient.

DISCHARGE PLANNING

Discharge planning is crucial to assure continuity of care, begins upon entry into the health-care situation and includes the expected discharge destination (e.g., home, skilled nursing facility, etc.). The nurse is committed to planning continuity of care between nursing personnel, between services within the care setting, and between the care setting and the community. The nurse may also be responsible for initiating/cooperating in referrals to other community services to provide needed direction for patient/family who are learning to facilitate recovery and promote wellness.

Some concerns associated with the identification of patient problems and the construction of the care plan include: What is the nurse's responsibility once a nursing diagnosis is made if the patient is discharged from care before all short-term outcomes are met and/or problems are resolved? Whose responsibility is it for follow-through for provision and evaluation of care once discharge has occurred? Who is responsible for monitoring patient progress toward long-term outcomes? Should this information be shared with the patient's admitting/primary physician or office nurse? Is the nurse who has made a nursing diagnosis responsible for follow-through to its resolution? Nationally, this issue is unresolved and patient outcomes may remain unmet. Ethically, it is the responsibility of the nursing community and the health-care industry to formulate policies that will promote optimal patient recovery and health maintenance.

CHAPTER 5

DOCUMENTATION OF CARE

Treatment planning begins upon the patient's admission to the health-care system with the identification of chief problems and the reason for admission using a variety of assessments. This treatment plan reflects evaluation and changes as applicable. All problems identified are addressed in the treatment plan. (If a problem is omitted, the reasons for this also must be documented.) The treatment plan is a legal document that records the sequence of events that occur while the patient is receiving care.

Once constructed, the care plan provides documentation of the planning process and serves as a framework/outline for the charting of administered care. The goals of the documentation system are to facilitate the quality of patient care, to ensure documentation of progress with regard to patient-focused outcomes, and to facilitate interdisciplinary consistency and communication of treatment goals and progress.

PROGRESS NOTES

Progress notes are an integral component of the overall medical record and should include all significant events that occur in the daily life of the patient. They should be written in a clear and objective fashion and in a manner that reflects progress toward expected measurable outcomes and the use of planned staff interventions.

Progress notes serve multiple functions, and any given note may be written to address one function more than the others. Thus it is important to recognize the seven major functions of progress notes:

1. Staff communication.
2. Legal documentation.
3. Evaluation.
4. Accreditation.
5. Training and supervision.
6. Reimbursement.
7. Relationship monitoring.

Staff Communication

Clearly, staff arriving on the next and subsequent shifts need to know what has been occurring with the patient during the current shift in order to make appropriate judgments regarding patient management. Co-worker to co-worker communication is the most obvious function of the progress notes, yet this is only a piece of the communication picture. Staff are in the unique position of being in contact with the patient for extended periods of time and a variety of situations. Their observations of patient behavior/response to therapy provide invaluable information to the physician or other provider who may only see the patient for a few minutes each day. Through this communication, it can be determined whether the patient's current expected measurable outcomes and interventions need to be eliminated or altered or whether the development of new outcomes or interventions are warranted.

Legal Documentation

In our increasingly litigious society, all aspects of the medical record, including the information contained in daily progress notes, may be important for legal documentation. For legal purposes, one must remember that if an event is not documented, it did not occur. Progress notes and flow sheets should therefore reflect implementation of the treatment plan as documentation that appropriate actions have been performed, precautions taken, and so forth. Both the implementation of interventions and the progress toward the expected measurable outcomes should be documented in the progress notes of the patient's medical record. These notations should also be specific as to date and time and should be signed by the person making the entry. Any errors in the document must be crossed out with one line so that they are still legible, identified by the author as an "error," and initialed. Whiteouts or cross-outs obliterating the information are not acceptable as they could be construed to mean that the individual or facility is trying to alter the facts.

Evaluation

Periodic review of the patient's progress and the effectiveness of the treatment plan is completed by the primary nurse and/or the treatment team. An evaluation of the patient's progress may be documented on the care plan or in the progress notes.

For the purposes of many outside reviews, the medical record should be written in a manner that facilitates an assessment of the care being given the patient. Progress notes should be written in a manner that reflects work on the patient's current desired measurable outcomes and interventions used to attain these outcomes. A person from outside of the facility should be able to read the notes and ascertain if the treatment plan is being implemented and if progress is being made on current desired measurable outcomes. The medical record should serve as a method of tracking the patient's response to treatment and consequently as a means for evaluating the quality of care provided.

Accreditation

For health-care facilities to be accredited by JCAHO and/or other accreditation and licensing agencies, the maintenance of a medical record is one of the most essential requirements. Standards state that the medical record be documented accurately and in a timely manner. Therefore, the importance of completing notes on schedule and in a manner that facilitates retrieval of data should be emphasized.

Training and Supervision

An often underestimated aspect of note writing is the value that such notes hold for training and supervision purposes. An experienced nurse's description of how s/he handled a complicated situation, a supervisor's analysis of the problems presented by a new admission, and a description of patterns noted in another patient's response to care are all examples of notes that provide training or supervision for the remainder of the staff. Supervisors also gain an impression of the employee's abilities through reading progress notes and may be able to isolate areas in which additional supervision or training/education would be beneficial.

Third-Party Reimbursement

Third-party reimbursers are insistent that the when, where, how, what, and who of services be clearly documented. An absence of such documentation may result in termination of funding for individual patients and therefore termination of treatment. The medical record is a primary source for maintaining the revenues as well as the patient's treatment. Progress notes must therefore document any significant observations that portray the patient's illness, treatment, and recovery as well as include data about medications and equipment used.

Relationship Monitoring

The relationship that exists between staff and patient is a key feature of treatment in any setting. In the psychiatric setting, many of the patient's pathologies are manifested in these relationships, and many indications of progress are first identified through the patient's ability to relate more positively and openly with staff. Thus, monitoring of the patient's relationships with the staff is essential.

Of no less importance are the patient's interpersonal relationships with peers. Many patients have experienced significant problems in their peer relationships before admission. Notes detailing the observed status of these relationships, how the patient interacts in group situations, competitive situations, in one-to-one situations, and so forth, have important clinical implications.

Also, the patient's relationship with significant others can impact general well-being, progress toward recovery, independence in self-care, and ultimately a successful transition to the home setting. In whatever area the patient is being cared for, whether general or psychiatric, observation and monitoring of these interactions are an important component of the nursing care plan.

DESCRIPTIVE NOTE WRITING

Clearly, there is a potentially wide readership for notes written in the medical record including co-workers, physicians, psychiatrists, psychologists, primary nurses, lawyers, judges, utilization reviewers, insurance personnel, surveyors, agency representatives, parents or guardians, and the patients themselves to name a few. Consideration of this wide readership helps to emphasize the need for clarity and precision in the progress notes.

Since progress notes have many purposes and many potential readers, their clarity and accurateness are essential. Persons should be able to read the notes and have an unambiguous picture of what occurred with the patient. The best way to ensure the clarity of progress notes is through the use of descriptive (or observational) statements. What follows is a comparison of judgmental language and descriptive language as well as guidelines for writing observation-based notes.

Judgmental Language

We are all aware of the possibilities for miscommunication that exist in ordinary conversations. The dangers of miscommunication may be even more prevalent when writing, where the opportunities for clarification that are present in face-to-face communication are absent. We all are habituated to speaking and writing in a manner that is judgmental, and therefore ambiguous, without our even being aware of it. Consider the following statements:

- "He asks for pain medication **too often.**"
- "He is **uncooperative** today."
- "She did a **good job** on her incentive spirometer today."
- "He is a **manipulative** patient."
- "The new patient is really **difficult.**"
- "He has a **poor** outlook."
- "She had a **bad attitude** about doing her physical therapy this morning."

The highlighted words in each of the above statements represent judgments, not facts. Without any elaboration or basis for comparison, each of the statements is a statement of opinion open to varying interpretations. There are five basic types of judgmental statements: statements that reference undefined periods of time; statements that reference undefined quantities; statements referring to qualities; statements that fail to specify any objective basis for the judgment made; and statements inferring clinical judgments.

Undefined Periods of Time

Statements that refer to undefined periods of time may contain words or phrases such as the following:

often	almost always	most of the time
rarely	frequently	now and then
seldom	occasionally	every so often

Use of these and similar phrases without clarification may leave the statement unclear and judgmental. How often, for example, is "every so often"? Every five minutes? Once an hour? Five times per shift? This is not to say that the staff member must time each and every interaction or occurrence.

Rather, one should be aware of the *potential* for confusion in these words. Ask the following questions: Does this note concern an event about which a more specific time relationship should be noted? If documenting for potential legal purposes (an injury, for example), specificity will be essential. For routine communication purposes, this may not be the case. Consider the following entry: "The patient was quiet for most of the shift today." The exact number of minutes during which the patient was or was not quiet is not necessary for reasonable, accurate communication to occur.

Undefined Quantities

Statements that refer to undefined quantities may use such words or phrases as the following:

some	enough	moderate	too much
a lot	more	very little	many

As with the statements that refer to undefined periods of time, each of these terms is open to interpretation. "A lot" of complaints to one person, for example, might mean five; to another it might mean twenty. As a rule, it is advisable to avoid undefined quantities.

Qualities

All descriptive adjectives applied to patients have the potential to belong in this category, since they may involve making subjective definitions beforehand. Of greatest concern, however, are words that could be called "semi-technical":

passive	irritating	incompetent
nervous	manipulative	over-protective
demanding	alcoholic	disturbed

Such words may have connotations in the health field beyond the scope of their ordinary definitions. Therefore, elaboration upon these qualities may be desirable. More common adjectives pose less of a problem and arouse less potential for misunderstanding:

friendly	unhappy	enthusiastic	proud
attentive	excited	bored	observant
aloof	apathetic	cheerful	happy

Finally, there are slang words, which besides being unclear, should not be contained in a professionally written note in any case. For example:

hyped-up	spaced-out	bummed	crazy
loose	pushy	cool	tanked-up

Failure to Provide an Objective Basis for Judgments

Some statements are self-evidently judgments, but offered without any objective basis. Such statements may cause the reader to ask, "How do you know that . . . ?"

This patient is improving.
This patient has the best attitude.
This patient likes to read.
This patient hates her roommate.

Inappropriate Use of Clinical Terminology

Although clearly implied by the above discussion of judgmental language, it is worth specifically noting that staff should avoid the use of clinical terminology in their notes. Unless one is qualified through education in nursing, occupational/physical therapy, social work, psychology, neurology, or other related fields and is additionally in a position requiring one to render clinical and diagnostic judgments, use of such terminology is subjective and possibly confusing to others. Examples of such inappropriate terms are given below:

passive-aggressive	hyperactive	noncompliant
narcissistic	borderline	incompetent
psychotic	schizophrenic	
depressed	displacement	

Descriptive Language

Descriptive language contains observations only and avoids statements that are evaluative or judgmental unless observational evidence can be presented to support the judgment. Remember that being able to actually observe the patient doing something was the criterion of a well-written measurable outcome. The situation is similar for observation-based progress notes; properly written objective statements refer to specific observable or measurable events. Descriptive statements contain measurable periods of time:

Ten times in 1 hour	Once
Every half hour	48 hours
Four times a day	15 minutes

Descriptive statements contain measurable quantities:

Twenty percent of the diet	All of the patients
Six out of eight	Completely saturated
None	5 ml

Descriptive statements provide a basis or rationale for qualities named in the note. You may have gotten the impression in the preceding section that you can never use adjectives in your notes. This is far from the case. In fact, you *should* give your impressions of the patient. Statements in which you note that the patient "seemed" or "appeared" to be exhibiting a certain physical/emotional state are inferential statements. These are a subset of descriptive statements in which you infer the patient's state based on your observations of his/her behavior and interactions, your knowledge of the patient's patterns, and the connections you make between behavior/affect and what has been happening during the illness. Such statements are often of great value. However, you should not allow your subjective impressions to stand alone, particularly if your observation involves some of the more "semi-technical" qualities noted earlier. You should also provide some reasons why you believed the patient was "improving," "demanding," "manipulative," and so forth:

- "The patient seemed upset by the news, as evidenced by the fact that she turned on her side and would not speak to caregivers."
- "Consistent with the pattern noted previously, the patient reacted to the change in his treatment by becoming upset and angry."
- "The patient appeared to be quite upset, verbally expressing her dismay at her inability to walk around the room."

Finally, when comparisons or judgments are made, a descriptive statement will state the source or basis of judgment:

- According to the patient's laboratory reports . . .
- Psychologic testing showed that . . .
- The other patient stated that . . .
- Judging by the fact that . . .

Note that whenever the source of a judgment is specified, the statement becomes a behavioral report. Because such a report can be observed, this type of statement is an observation and is therefore descriptive. For example, consider the difference between the following two statements:

1. The patient is experiencing anxiety.
2. The physician said that "the patient is experiencing anxiety."

The first statement is clearly judgmental because of the undefined phrase "experiencing anxiety." The second, however, is an observable event. Obviously (although the physician may be wrong) it is an objective fact that s/he said that the patient is experiencing anxiety. It may help to think of such statements as quotations. *What* the physician said does not influence our ability to observe him/her saying it and objectively report that observation.

Finally, the nurse can chart observations in a nonjudgmental manner:

"The patient displayed increased anxiety, pacing about the room, wringing his hands."

Comparison of Judgmental and Behavioral Notes

The important thing to observe about judgmental statements is that they may be translated into more precise terms. A staff member's assertion that "The patient did pretty well today," for example, might boil down to "The patient followed directions for drawing up and administering her insulin without any mistakes." Below are some other examples of how judgmental statements may be interpreted more objectively:

a. The meeting with the physical therapist did not go very well.
b. The patient stated she could not do the exercises, that were to be started today.

a. The patient had a bad attitude today.
b. The patient argued with staff five times during the shift.

a. The patient became aggressive.
b. The patient clenched his fists and yelled to the nurse, "I'd like to hit you." He then hit the wall twice with his fist.

a. The patient would not follow directions.
b. The patient drank a glass of water 30 minutes before his scheduled surgery.

a. The patient ate poorly.
b. The patient ate one third of her lunch (all of the broccoli and corn, no meat) and drank 50 cc of apple juice.

As demonstrated by these examples, it often takes a bit more thought to write a note that is objectively descriptive. However, the benefits in clarity of communication make the effort essential for the many purposes of progress notes.

Content of Note/Entry

The term *progress note* indicates that the patient's *progress* is to be documented along with the implementation of the treatment plan. Contents should be as specific and exact as possible.

For communication purposes, it is important to record in the progress notes any information that is of importance to nurses that will be working the oncoming shifts as well as observations that may be significant for professional staff. In *The Other 23 Hours*, James K. Whittaker stresses the importance of documenting critical incidents in the patient's treatment. He describes four broad types of critical incidents:

1. Unsettled or unclear problems or "issues" that should be dealt with by a nurse on the oncoming shift, the supervisor, or the physician.
2. Noteworthy incidents or interviews involving the patient that would benefit from a more detailed recording.
3. Other pertinent data such as notes on phone calls, home visits, and life space interview summaries.
4. Additional critical incident criteria . . . "which might include seemingly significant or revealing statements made by the patient, an insight you have into a patient's patterns of behavior, etc."

Critical incident reporting regarding patient injuries, the use of any special treatment procedure, or other major events such as episodes of pain, respiratory distress, panic attacks, medication reactions, or suicidal comments should always be documented in the progress notes and should be especially precise. The use of restraints, for example, should always be noted in the progress notes. Moreover, the exact time the procedure was initiated, whether any injuries resulted, and so forth, should be documented. In cases such as this, it is also necessary to document what led up to the situation, how staff and other participants reacted, what less restrictive measures were tried, and any significant observations regarding the incident.

Other areas of concern that enhance accurate communication are the use of correct grammar and spelling, legible writing, and the use of nonerasable ink. Avoiding the repetition of data when possible promotes clarity of documentation. Using the patient's name "Mary Jones" rather than the vague term "patient" can avoid problems if parts of the record become separated. Having a name noted can identify the proper chart and prevent problems of misidentification. Abbreviations should be used with caution or avoided in most instances. They can be misleading or easily misinterpreted, resulting in misunderstandings and errors with serious consequences. Some institutions have approved certain abbreviations to be used within the institution and provide a list that identifies the correct meaning.

Format of Note/Entry

There are several charting formats currently used for documentation. These include (1) block notes with a single entry covering an entire shift (e.g., 7 AM–3 PM), (2) narrative timed notes (e.g., 8:30 AM, Ate breakfast well), and (3) the problem-oriented record system (POMR or PORS) using SOAP/SOAPIER approach, to name a few. While the third format can provide thorough documentation, it requires that the entries be tied to a problem and may not always promote nursing process documentation.

The Focus system has been designed to encourage viewing the patient from a positive perspective rather than a negative one by using precise documentation to record the nursing process. Charting focuses on nursing concerns, with the focal point being nursing issues identified through the assessment phase of the nursing process. A *Focus* is usually a patient problem/concern or nursing diagnosis, but is *not* a medical diagnosis or a nursing task/treatment (e.g., wound care, Foley catheter insertion, tube feeding). Choosing the appropriate focus for a specific patient will depend on the planned content of the note, for whom the note is written, and how the information can be most clearly communicated. Recording of assessment, interventions, and evaluation in a Data, Action, and Response (DAR) format facilitates following what is happening to the patient at any given moment. Thus, the four components of this charting system are:

1. Focus: nursing diagnosis, patient problem/concern.
2. Data: subjective/objective information describing and/or supporting the Focus.
3. Action: immediate/future nursing actions based on assessment and consistent with/complementary to the goals and nursing action recorded in the patient care plan.
4. Response: describes the effects of interventions and whether or not the goal was met.

Although each note should have a Focus, the three components of Data, Action, and Response may not be addressed in each entry.

Example:

Time	Focus	D = Data A = Action R = Response		Date: May 15, 1989
0800	Constipation	D	c/o discomfort, feeling of fullness. States "no BM for three days." Auscultation of abdomen reveals dullness, decreased bowel sounds; and presence of distention.	
		A	Dietary regimen, fluid in-	

			take, and previous pattern reviewed. Encourage Ms. Rogers to maintain high-fiber/bulk diet and to increase intake of fluids (including juices) to 2000 cc/day. Promote increased activity. Dr. Smith notified. Fleet's enema given.
0930	Constipation	R	Results of enema: hard, formed stool expelled. Ms. Rogers states "feels more comfortable." Abdomen softer, bowel sounds clear.

Summary

Use of clear documentation for planning patient care helps the nurse to individualize patient care, set priorities, and provide a picture of what has happened and what is happening to promote continuity of care as well as ongoing evaluation. This reinforces each person's accountability and responsibility for using nursing process. As these skills are improved, time will be saved by the consistent use of a system that focuses on specific issues. This documentation of professional nursing care can also help in meeting legal and accreditation requirements without having to spend additional time gathering information together when these occasions arise.

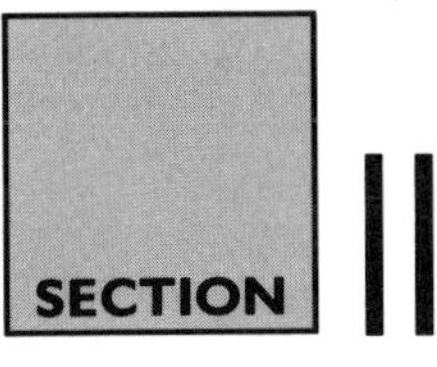

II

SEVEN PATIENT SITUATION CARE PLAN PROTOTYPES

This section takes theory and puts it into practice. It represents application of the nursing process and shows how the components (assessment, problem identification, planning, intervention, and evaluation) are used in the development of a care plan. Patient problem statements (nursing diagnoses) are formulated using *related to* and *evidenced by* information. Goals are created with appropriate time lines (measurable outcomes).

Although not included in a regular care plan, *rationale* has been provided in this book to help the nurse/student learn and understand why a particular intervention has been chosen.

MEDICAL CARE PLAN: ANGINA

Mr. N.K., a 61-year-old man, is admitted to the medical unit with a diagnosis of unstable angina. He has had two myocardial infarctions and underwent triple coronary bypass surgery 14 years ago.

ADMITTING PHYSICIAN'S ORDERS

CBC, chemistry profile, cardiac enzymes, liver profile, digoxin level, urinalysis in AM.
Chest x-ray/ECG in AM.
Schedule exercise thallium stress test for 1/10, AM.
Telemetry monitoring, document dysrhythmias.
Digoxin 0.25 mg PO noon daily; hold if rate less than 50.
Nitroglycerin 0.15 mg SL at bedside.
Procardia 20 mg qid.
Inderal 40 mg qid.
NitroDur 2 in q 12 h.
Enteric-coated ASA 5 gr each AM and PM.
Low cholesterol/low sodium diet. Dietitian to instruct.
Begin in-house graduated rehabilitation program, level I. Advance daily as tolerated.

NURSING HISTORY AND ASSESSMENT

Name: N.K. Informant: Patient
Reliability (scale 1–4): 4
Age: 61 Sex: Male
DOB: 10/12/23 Race: Caucasian
Admission date: 1/8/85 Time: 1700
From: Home
Family member/significant other(s): A.K. (wife)

ACTIVITY/REST

Subjective

Sleep: Hours: 6–8 hr/night
Naps: -0- Aids: -0-
Insomnia: Occasional Related to: Problems at work
Rested on awakening: "More or less"
Occupation: Owner, floor covering company
Usual activities/hobbies: Reading mystery/detective novels, woodworking—but not recently
Leisure time activities: "Watch TV news; 1 or 2 times per month my wife and I take a Sunday drive"
Limitations imposed by illness: Chest pain, gets short of breath, e.g., climbing full flight of stairs or walking 3–4 blocks at a brisk pace

Objective

Observed response to activity: No angina presently
Mental status: Alert, oriented, calm
Muscle mass/tone: Fair Posture: Good
ROM: Good
Strength: (scale 0–4) R leg 2+/L Leg 3+

CIRCULATION

Subjective

Reports history of high BP before CVA in 1982
Heart trouble: MI × 2, 1960, 1969; CABG × 3 vessels, 1971; CHF, 1970
Ankle edema/slow healing: -0-

Claudication: Relieved by transluminal angioplasty R femoral artery, 1980
Numbness: Occasional R leg, since angioplasty
Tingling: Same
Cough/character of sputum: -0-
Change in frequency/amount of urine: Occasional nocturia, TUR for BPH, 1980

Objective:

BP: R: Sit 150/80 Lying: 138/78
Stand: 164/80
L: Sit 148/80 Lying: 138/70
Stand: 164/80
Pulse pressure: 50–70 Auscultatory gap: -0-
Pulses: Carotid: 3+/equal Radial: 3+/equal
Femoral: 3+/equal Popliteal: 2+/equal
Post-tibial: R 1+/L 2+
Dorsalis pedis: R 1+/L 2+
Cardiac: PMI fifth intercostal space, medial to L midclavicular line
Thrill/Heaves: -0-
Heart sounds: $S_1 - S_2$ normal Rate: 88 no pulse deficit
Rhythm: regular Quality: Normal
Friction rub/murmur: -0-
Breath sounds: Clear and equal bilaterally
Vascular bruit: deferred Jugular vein distention: -0-
Capillary refill: R leg > 3 sec Temperature of extremities: Legs cool
Homan's sign: -0- History of R calf thrombophlebitis, 1971
Distribution and quality of hair: Lack of hair below midshin R leg
Color: Skin: Pale/no cyanosis Mucous membranes/lips: Pink
Nailbeds: Pale, blanch well
Conjunctiva: Clear
Sclera: White

EGO INTEGRITY

Subjective

Report of stress factors: "Lots of stress at work"
Ways of handling stress: "I keep on my employees so the work gets done.
At home I have some Scotch, watch the news, and put my feet up."
Financial concerns: Trying to sell business so he can retire
Cultural factors: Urban; "American, mixed background/strong German"
Religion: Practicing Catholic
Lifestyle/changes: Upper middle class/approaching retirement
Feelings of helplessness: "No, I think I'm more frustrated"

Objective

Emotional status: Calm, quiet, watchful.
Other (specify): Considers himself "well" in spite of medical history and present angina
Observed physiologic response(s): Controlled with arms/legs crossed

ELIMINATION

Subjective

Usual bowel pattern: Every evening
Last BM: Last PM Character of stool: Soft/formed
Bleeding/hemorrhoids: -0- Diarrhea: -0-
Constipation: occasional
Laxative used: MOM on rare occasions.

Pain/burning/difficulty with urination?: Occasional episodes of frequency noted since TUR.
Incontinence: -0- Character of urine: Clear/yellow

Objective

Abdomen: Tender: -0- Soft/firm: Soft
Palpable Mass: -0-
Bowel sounds: Active all 4 quadrants Size/girth: Not measured
Palpate bladder: Not palpable

FOOD/FLUID

Subjective

Diet (type): Low fat, low sodium
Dietary pattern: Skips lunch; 5–6 cups coffee/day.
Last meal/intake: Breakfast; toast, cereal, coffee
Loss of appetite: -0- Nausea/vomiting: -0-
Heartburn/indigestion: Occasional R/T: spicy food, caffeinated coffee
Relieved by: Antacid tablets
Allergy/food intolerance: -0-
Chewing/swallowing problems: -0- Dentures (upper/lower): -0-
Usual wt: 155 lb Changes in weight; Increased 10 lb this year
Diuretic therapy: Hydrodiuril daily.

Objective

Current Wt: 165 lb Ht: 5′5″
Body build: Stocky
Skin turgor: Good Mucous membranes: Moist
Hernia/masses: -0-

Edema/jugular distention: -0-
Condition of teeth/gums: Good hygiene
Halitosis: -0-
Appearance of tongue: Midline, moist Mucous membranes: Pink/intact
Bowel sounds: Active all 4 quadrants
Breath sounds: Normal/clear

HYGIENE

Subjective

Activities of daily living: Independent in all areas

Objective

General appearance: Well-groomed, hair combed, nails trimmed

NEUROSENSORY

Subjective

Fainting spells/dizziness: At time of TIAs
Headaches: "Occasionally when I'm overstressed"
Seizures: -0- Tingling/numbness: -0-
Weakness (location): R sided, resolved a few days after CVA
Stroke: CVA 1982; TIA 1981, 1982, no residual effects
Eyes/vision loss: Nearsighted Glaucoma: -0-
Cataract: -0-
Ears/hearing loss: -0-
Nose: Epistaxis -0- Sense of smell: No complaints/not tested

Objective

Memory recent/remote: Both clear/accurate
Mental status: Alert and oriented to time, place, and person.
Delusions: -0- Hallucinations: -0-
Affect: Appropriate to context of situation.
Glasses: Yes Contacts: No Pupil reaction: PERL
Facial droop: -0-
Swallowing: No difficulty noted
Handgrip/release: Strong/equal
Speech: Clear/intelligible

PAIN/COMFORT

Subjective

Location: Substernal, L shoulder/arm
Frequency: approximately 4 times per wk
Intensity (scale 1–10): 6–8
Quality: Burning/squeezing
Duration: ≥3–5 minutes Radiation: Sometimes into L arm
Precipitating factors: Exercise and stressful situation, e.g., climbing flight of stairs, walking 3–4 blocks, employee/customer problems
How relieved: Rest with feet elevated and eyes closed; Nitro doesn't seem to help

Objective

Pain free at the moment; no observation made

RESPIRATION

Subjective

Dyspnea/related to: Exertion or with pain
Cough/productive: Rare Emphysema: -0-

Bronchitis: -0-
Asthma: -0- Smoker: no Use of respiratory aids: -0-

Objective

Respiratory rate: 16 Depth: Deep/equal bilaterally
Auscultation: Breath sounds equal bilaterally; no crackles/rhonchi
Use of accessory muscles: -0- Nasal flaring: -0-
Cyanosis: -0- Clubbing of fingers: -0-
Sputum characteristics: -0-
Mentation/restlessness: Alert/oriented/calm

SAFETY

Subjective

Allergies/sensitivity: Iodine dye
Reaction: Hives
History of sexually transmitted disease: -0-
Blood transfusions: 14 When: CABG, 1971
Reaction: -0-
History of accidental injuries: -0-
Fractures/dislocations: -0- Arthritis/unstable joints: -0-
Back problems: -0- Changes in moles: -0-
Prostheses: -0- Ambulatory devices: -0-
Vision impaired: Wears glasses Hearing impaired: -0-

Objective

Temperature: 97.6°F PO
Skin integrity: Intact Rashes: -0-

Sores: -0- Bruises: -0-
Scars: Surgical scars midline chest, both legs.
Strength (general): Adequate for age; legs weaker than arms
Muscle tone: Fair ROM: Normal
Gait: Normal
Paresthesia/Paralysis: -0-

SEXUALITY Male:

Subjective

Sexual concerns: "Too old to think about sex very much"
Penile discharge: -0- Prostate disorder: BPH and TUR, 1980
Vasectomy: -0- Practice self-exam: Breast/testicles: No
Use of condoms: No
Last proctoscopic exam: 1984 Prostate exam: 6/84

Objective

Exam: Breast: No masses noted during auscultation/palpation
Testicles: Deferred Prostate: Deferred

SOCIAL INTERACTION

Subjective

Relationship status: Married
Years in relationship: 34
Living with: Wife
Extended family: Two grown sons living out of state

Other support persons: "None unless you count my secretary"
Role: Husband/father
Report of problems: "None except financial worries"
Coping behaviors: "Just deal with what has to be done; used to get away and play golf when I could"
Frequency of social contacts: "Too busy to socalize regularly"

Objective

Verbal/nonverbal communication with family/significant other(s): Patient turns to wife for agreement after answering nurse's questions
Family interaction patterns: Patient and wife reading/watching TV news together and discussing day's events in relaxed manner before interview

TEACHING/LEARNING

Subjective

Dominant language: English
Level of education: 2 yr college/business management
Health beliefs/practices: "I try to follow my doctor's advice"
Special health-care practices: None
Familial risk factors: (Indicate relationship)
Cancer: Father died at 54, colon CA
Kidney disease: -0-
Heart disease: Mother died at 72, CHF
Strokes: -0- High BP: -0-

Diabetes: -0- Tuberculosis: -0-
Epilepsy: -0- Mental illness: -0-

Routine medications as stated by patient:

Drug	*Dose:*	*Schedule:*	*Time/last dose:*
Inderal	10 mg	8-1-6-9	1 PM
Digoxin	0.25 mg	8 AM daily	8 AM
Nitropaste	1.5 in	8 AM–8 PM	8 AM
Hydrodiuril	50 mg	8 AM daily	8 AM
Procardia	20 mg	8-1-6-9	1 PM
Nitro	0.15 mg 1–2 tabs	prn pain	None today

Does patient take medications regularly?: Usually faithful

Does patient notice any ill effects from medications?: "Can't tell"

Nonprescription (OTC) drugs: Occasional ASA

Use of alcohol (amount/frequency): 1–2 drinks at night

Admitting diagnosis (physician): Unstable angina

Reason for hospitalization (patient): "Find out why my medicines aren't controlling my chest pain"

History of current complaint: "Chest pains increasing in frequency, traveling to my left shoulder and arm with exercise and at work"

Other relevant illness and/or previous hospitalizations/surgeries:

Numerous hospitalizations (documented elsewhere in this history)

Last hospitalized 3 years ago, TIA

Patient expectations of this hospitalization? "Help me find out if I should retire, and see if anything can be done about this chest pain"

Evidence of failure to improve: Yes, recurring chest pain

Last physical exam: 6 months ago

DISCHARGE CONSIDERATIONS

Date data obtained: 1/8/85
Anticipated date of discharge: 1/11/85
Resources available: Persons: Wife Financial: "Adequate for now," has health insurance
Does not anticipate any need for post-discharge assistance or changes in living situation

MEDICAL/SURGICAL CARE PLAN: ANGINA

PATIENT PROBLEM STATEMENT/ FOCUS (NURSING DIAGNOSIS)

Activity intolerance related to interruption/reduction of cardiac blood flow evidenced by chest pain and dyspnea with exertion/stress.

PATIENT OUTCOMES/ EVALUATION CRITERIA

Short-term:

- Displays increased activity level with reduced frequency/severity of pain and dyspnea, within 48 hours (1500 1/10).

Long-term:

- Maintains desired activity level free of pain/dyspnea within 3 weeks (1/29/85).

Actions/Interventions	Rationale
Assess chest pain: Identify precipitating/ relieving factors. Note time, duration, intensity (1–10).	Assists in differentiating angina from other sources of pain, e.g., intercostal/ chest wall pain or impending MI. *Note:* pain precipitated by climbing stairs, lasting from a few seconds to minutes, rated 5 or greater on intensity scale, and relieved by rest is likely angina related to myocardial ischemia.

Actions/Interventions	Rationale
Monitor vital signs:	
Heart rate:	Can increase or decrease in response to ischemia/pain, anxiety.
Heart rhythm:	Coronary vasospasm with transient ischemia can cause changes in electrical conduction.
Heart sounds:	Presence of S_4 during angina indicative of ischemia. Should resolve following administration of nitroglycerin.
Blood pressure:	May increase in response to pain, unless cardiac decompensation is severe.
Respirations:	Dyspnea with cyanosis associated with severe angina may indicate reduced cardiac output or impending infarction.
Encourage N.K. to be up and to participate in supervised activities.	Provides safe environment to identify precipitating factors and degree of physiologic involvement.

Begin in-patient cardiac exercise program at level I, and increase daily as tolerated.

May be useful in identifying level at which pain occurs. Graduated level of reconditioning/ strength building to be continued post-discharge.

Monitor cardiac rhythm continuously by telemetry: Document baseline rhythm, dysrhythmias.

Allows patient to be active. Identifies rhythm disturbances related to angina episodes and/or activity.

Administer medications:

Procardia (Nifedepine) 20 mg qid (0800–1300–1800 2200);

Calcium blocking agent with antianginal effects related to calcium flux alterations on cardiac muscle.

Digoxin 0.25 mg daily (1200) Document apical/radial 60-second heart rate; hold if rate below 50;

Inotropic agent that strengthens cardiac contraction. Used for long-term management of CHF, and chronic ischemic heart disease. Drug may be withheld dependent on heart rate as defined by physician.

Inderol 40 mg qid

Beta-blocking agent

Actions/Interventions	Rationale
with food (0800–1300–1800–2200);	with antianginal, antihypertensive, and antiarrythmic properties.
Nitro-Dur (paste) 2 in q 12 hr, (0800–2000);	Nitrate with vasodilator properties for treatment of chronic ischemic heart disease.
Enteric-coated ASA gr 5, AM/PM (0800–2000).	Analgesic with mild anticoagulant effects may be used to treat headache, side effects of nitrates, and/or prophylactic use in patient with previously documented TIA/MI. Enteric coating reduces risk of gastric irritation. risk of gastric irritation.
Nitroglycerin gr 1/150 SL prn.	Rapid-acting nitrate/vasodilator that improves coronary blood flow to relieve/prevent episodic pain.
Evaluate response to drug therapy. Monitor for side effects.	Drug choice/dosage is dependent on individual response and/or presence of undesired side effects.

Administer oxygen 2–3 L/m via nasal cannula prn for severe or unrelieved chest pain.	Ischemic pain may be relieved by supplemental oxygen if other measures not effective.
Provide pretest procedure information/purpose about exercise Thallium stress test.	Will be better prepared psychologically for the physical discomfort he could experience during treadmill time and understand that its purpose is to assess physical limitation to exertion in preparation for cardiac rehabilitation program, or possible alteration in lifestyle.

PATIENT PROBLEM STATEMENT/ FOCUS (NURSING DIAGNOSIS)

Tissue perfusion, altered: peripheral related to interruption/alteration of both venous and arterial flow to legs (atherosclerotic/thromboembolic incident) evidenced by residual diminished pulse, cool skin temperature and demarcation hair midcalf right leg.

PATIENT OUTCOMES/ EVALUATION CRITERIA

Short-term:
- Identifies individual risk/safety factors within 48 hours (1500 1/10).

Long-term:
- Reports absence of signs/symptoms of further impairment of circulation to lower extremities (ongoing).

Actions/Interventions:	Rationale:
Assess presence/ quality of femoral, popliteal, tibial, pedal pulses.	Note deviation from baseline. (Right pedal pulse documented to be less than left, related to previous transluminal angioplasty.)
Note skin temperature/color. Observe toenail beds for capillary refill.	Right leg documented cool and pale related to previous impairment. Slow capillary refill indicates present but impaired circulation.
Evaluate tolerance to activity/walking. Measure distance; report leg discomfort.	Patient being prepared for post-discharge cardiac rehabilitation program.

Document sudden changes.	Indicative of acute circulatory impairment requiring intervention.
Review individual symptoms and changes indicating need for medical evaluation.	Increases patient awareness and provides opportunity for prompt intervention.
Discuss proper foot/skin care and avoidance of restrictive clothing.	Reduces risk of complications/increased circulatory impairment.

PATIENT PROBLEM STATEMENT/ FOCUS (NURSING DIAGNOSIS)

Knowledge deficit related to lack of understanding of complexities of medical condition/therapies evidenced by request for information about drug regimen, specific actions to deal with anginal episodes, and preparation for lifestyle changes (retirement).

PATIENT OUTCOMES/ EVALUATION CRITERIA

Short-term:

- Correctly identifies problems requiring immediate medical attention within 24 hours (1500 1/9).
- Verbalizes knowledge/understanding of chronic angina/peripheral vascular disease and therapy regimen within 48 hours (1500 1/10).

- Demonstrates techniques/behaviors to manage stress within 48 hours (1500 1/10).

  Long-term:
- Displays no preventable complications (ongoing).

Actions/Interventions	Rationale
Determine level of knowledge regarding recurrent angina with medical intervention.	Understanding that surgical intervention is not the first option is important to acceptance of other alternatives of care.
Identify motivating factors for learning.	Provides direction for teaching/learning.
Determine N.K.'s most urgent need from N.K's/wife's and nurse's viewpoint.	Provides priority for planning direction, e.g., N.K. desires pain management, believing that pain is interfering with needed/desired lifestyle. He also wants to reduce work stressors and increase his exercise tolerance. Wife just wants him to relax and be well. Nurse is concerned about proper/safe administration of medications, believing that N.K. needs guidelines for

	safe drug administration as well as reason (motive) for continuity of regimen.
Coordinate written information from all disciplines on discharge plan of care.	Helpful for N.K./wife to refer to later for reinforcement.
Involve N.K./wife in team and group teaching/support sessions (1100 1/9 and 1/10). Use audiovisual materials and questions/dialogue.	Can achieve learning/support from group. Audiovisual materials may provide information that patient has been reluctant to ask about.
Arrange instruction session by dietitian on low fat, low sodium diet.	Can work with patient's likes/dislikes/habits and wife's cooking style to initiate workable eating plan to enable patient to lose about 10 lb.
Identify/discuss blocks to success of dietary plan and ways to cooperate.	Knowing blocks to success allows for planning ways to avoid them.
Provide positive reinforcement.	Past adherence to low fat/sodium diet has been successful enough to enable him to discontinue

Actions/Interventions	Rationale
	taking antilipid drug, Atromid.
Review/assess prior teaching regarding medications: indications, usual effect, dose, time, side effects.	Provides opportunity to reinforce positive behaviors, identify misconceptions, redirect behaviors for optimal benefit.
Reinforce/discuss safety factors associated with present drug therapy:	Discussion provides verbalization of patient's understanding and clues to possible cooperation/lack of cooperation with plan.
Nitroglycerin: May take q 5 minutes × 3 during angina attacks;	Rapid, short acting. Safe to repeat several times.
May take before anticipated stress	Prophylactic action.
Wet tablet with saliva and hold under tongue, (subliminal and not to be chewed or swallowed whole);	Provides for optimal and timely absorption of medication.
Store in cool/dark place in closed container with cotton removed.	Drug is light sensitive and cotton absorbs drug, reducing potency over time.

Replace supply every 3 months;	
May experience side effects of headache/ flushing. These are normal and should gradually decrease;	Aspirin or Tylenol may be used if discomfort keeps patient from using nitroglycerin.
Report change in anginal pattern or failure to obtain pain relief.	May reflect deterioration or condition unrelated to cardiac status.
Procardia: Notify doctor of dizziness, weakness, syncope.	Interacts with Inderal. May reduce blood pressure or cause heart failure (rare).
Digoxin: Count pulse for 60 seconds before taking drug. Do not take drug before talking with doctor if heart rate less than 50;	Prevents likelihood of drug toxicity in presence of heart failure.
Report extreme fatigue, weakness, "yellow halos," blurred vision.	Signs/symptoms of digitalis toxicity.
Inderal: Take with food.	Increases absorption.
Instruct in relaxation/ stress management techniques, e.g., breathing exercises,	History reflects relationship of angina and stress. Techniques have

Actions/Interventions	Rationale
walking, biofeedback, tapes, etc., matched to individual needs.	positive physiological effects, e.g., decreased breathing, heart rate, BP.

CRITICAL CARE SITUATION: MULTIPLE TRAUMA

B.R., a 37-year-old iron worker is admitted to the hospital following an industrial accident. A large steel girder fell 10 feet from a crane, knocked B.R. to the floor, and pinned him down for several minutes before he could be freed. Upon admission to the Emergency Room, he presented with the following symptoms:

> BP was 80/40; respirations were 40 and shallow; and pulse was 130, and thready. Skin was cool, pale, and diaphoretic. Pupils were equal and reactive to light (PERL). The patient was stuporous, but responded to painful stimuli by grimacing, moaning and by answering to his name. Bystanders report that he was alert at the scene. A large hematoma was noted on his left anterior thigh; toes were pale and cool; and pedal pulse was diminished. The abdomen was distended, tense, and quiet; numerous ecchymotic areas and abrasions were noted on his abdomen and chest. Breath sounds were clear and equal with diminished bases. Chest movement was shallow, symmetrical, and splinting. Heart sounds were $S_1 - S_2$ regular.

Diagnostic Studies Done in E.R.

CBC: Hgb: 10.1, Hct: 38%.
Urinalysis: 10–15 RBC; otherwise negative.
Chem. profile: negative.
X-rays: Chest, fractures of left 9th, 10th, and 11th ribs; L leg negative for fracture, suggestive of soft-tissue injury; pelvis, linear fracture of left ileum.
Abdominal tap/lavage: Positive for blood.

Initial Treatment

An arterial line was placed in right radial artery and an indwelling catheter was inserted. A subclavian intravenous line was placed, and Lactated Ringer's infusion was given at a rapid rate while awaiting completion of type and crossmatch.

The patient was taken to surgery for abdominal exploration where a splenectomy was performed, and approximately 1500 cc of blood was removed from the abdominal cavity. The intestine was found to be intact. While in surgery, blood pressure remained low and the patient received two units whole blood. He was then admitted to the surgical intensive care unit.

ADMITTING PHYSICIAN'S ORDERS

VS q 15–30 minutes until stable; CVP q 1 hr.
Hourly urine output. Report u/o <35 cc/hr × 2 hr.
IV: D5 1/2 NS at 150 cc/hr.
1 unit packed cells now. Repeat H & H in 6 hr.
ABG's upon admission to unit and repeat in AM.
Electrolytes, CBC, chest x-ray in AM.
M.S. 2–4 mg IV q hr prn pain.
Cefotaxime 1 gm IVPB q 4 hr.
O_2 4 L per cannula.
Incentive spirometer q 4 hr.
Salem NG to intermittent suction; irrigate with NS prn.
May turn side to side with support.
Apply Rib belt.
Change surgical dressing prn.
Ice pack to L thigh × 48 hr. Check pulses/sensation L leg q 1 hr × 6 then q 2 hr. Report any decrease in circulation/sensation.

NURSING HISTORY AND ASSESSMENT

Name: B.R. Informant: Wife 11/6 and self 11/7
Age: 37 DOB: 3/17/50 Sex: Male
Race: Caucasian Admission date: 11/6/87
Time: 5:15 PM From: OR Family member/significant other(s): wife

ACTIVITY/REST

Subjective (11/6)

Sleep: Hours: 7–8 hr/night Naps: -0-
Aids: -0- Insomnia: Rare
Usual activities/hobbies: Watches TV, sports
Leisure-time activities: Bowling in winter, softball in summer
Limitations imposed by illness: 6–8 weeks convalescence anticipated
Occupation: Iron worker

Objective (11/6)

Observed response to activity: Deferred (on bedrest)
Mental status: Sedated
Muscle mass/tone: Muscular/firm
Equality of extremities: L arm/leg weaker (soft-tissue injuries, rib fractures)
Posture: Supine Tremors/deformity: -0-
ROM: R arm/leg, full; pain limits L shoulder/hip.
Strength: R hand slightly weaker (arterial line present).

CIRCULATION

Subjective (11/6)

History of elevated BP: -0- Heart trouble: -0-
Ankle edema: -0-

Extremities: Numbness/tingling: -0-
Claudication: -0-   Slow healing: -0-
Cough/character of sputum: -0-
Change in frequency/amount of urine: -0-

Objective (11/6)

BP: R: Sit: Deferred
Lying: 98/64   Stand: Deferred
L: Sit: Deferred
Lying: 90/60   Stand: Deferred
Pulse pressure: 30–34   Auscultatory gap: -0-
Pulse: Apical: 120, S_1/S_2, no murmurs/rub
PMI: Normal
Radial: 120   Quality: 2+
Rhythm: regular
Breath sounds: Few crackles
Jugular vein distention: -0-
Peripheral pulses: Diminished left popliteal and pedal 1+ each, right side 2+
Capillary refill: >5 seconds L toes, <5 seconds R toes
Temperature of extremities: L foot cooler than right
Homan's sign: -0-   Distribution and quality of hair: To toes/equal
Color: Skin: Pale
Mucous membranes/lips: Pale pink
Nailbeds: Pale to slightly dusky

EGO INTEGRITY

Subjective (11/7)

Report of stress factors: "I worried about getting laid off before accident, now I guess it will happen for sure"

Ways of handling stress: "A few beers, bowling, or going to batting cage"
Financial concerns: "Have good sick leave; Workmen's Compensation will pay for this"
Relationship status: Married
Cultural factors: Laborer/parents were Polish immigrants
Religion: Protestant/non-practicing
Lifestyle: Middle income/no recent changes
Believes he's usually in control of life unless economy results in layoff.

Objective (11/6)

Emotional status: Anxious, restive
Other (specify): Experiencing pain
Observed physiologic response(s): Heart rate 120; Respirations 28; Facial grimacing/tension.

ELIMINATION

Subjective (11/7)

Last BM: 11/6 AM Character of stool: Soft/brown
Bleeding: No Diarrhea: No
Constipation: No Laxative used: None
Pain/burning/difficulty with urination: No
Incontinence: No
Usual character of urine: Clear/yellow

Objective (11/6)

Abdomen tender: Yes Soft/firm: Firm
Palpable mass: -0-
Bowel sounds: Absent postoperatively
Size/girth: Deferred

Hemorrhoids: -0-
Urine: Dark amber, hazy per indwelling catheter, few RBCs noted on urinalysis 11/6.

FOOD/FLUID

Subjective (11/7)

Loss of appetite: -0- Mastication problems/ swallowing: -0-
Dentures: -0- Dietary pattern: 3 meals, 4 cups coffee
Special diet (type): Regular
Nausea/vomiting: Currently nauseated
Heartburn (food intolerance): Occasional to spicy food
Changes in weight: -0- Diuretic therapy: N/A
Last meal/intake: Lunch yesterday: 2 meat sandwiches, tomato soup, apple, chocolate cookies, coffee

Objective (11/6)

Wt: admission 180 lb Ht: 6′ Skin turgor: Fair
Edema: -0- Jugular distention: -0-
Appearance of tongue: Midline, dry, coated
Mucous membranes: Pale, dry
Condition of teeth/gums: Good, no gum problems noted
Halitosis: -0-
Breath sounds: Lungs clear; RR 28

HYGIENE

Subjective (11/6)

Activities of daily living: Has been independent—will need assistance in some areas at this time (NANDA scale: 0–4)

Mobility: 3 Feeding: 2 Dressing: N/A
Toileting: 1 Hygiene: 1

Objective (11/6)

General appearance: Tan; calloused hands with dirt/grease under nails; hair cut short; trimmed moustache
Body odor: -0- Presence of vermin: -0-

NEUROSENSORY

Subjective (11/7)

Fainting spells/dizziness: "Once with flu"
Stroke/Seizures: -0-
Weakness/tingling: -0- Numbness: "Left foot feels asleep"
Eyes/vision loss: Nearsighted/exam 10 months ago
Glaucoma/cataract: -0- Ears: Hearing loss: -0-
Nose: Epistaxis: -0- Sense of smell: "No problems"

Objective (11/6)

Mental status: Sedated, arouses easily, oriented to person, place.
Delusions/hallucinations: -0-
Affect: Apprehensive
Glasses: Yes Contacts: -0-
Pupil reaction: PERL Size: 4 mm decreased briskly to 3 mm
Hand grip/release: (R) slightly weaker (arterial line)
Hearing aid: No Speech: Mumbled but appropriate

PAIN/COMFORT

Subjective (11/6)

Location: Left hip, pelvis, abdomen, rib cage
Intensity (Scale 1–10): 10
Quality: Severe Duration: Constant, medication helps
Radiation: Ribs to back, all of L leg.
Precipitating factors: Injuries, movement
How relieved: Morphine

Objective (11/6)

Facial grimacing: Yes Guarding affected areas: Yes
Narrowed focus: Yes
Other: Splinting and somewhat limited chest expansion

RESPIRATION

Subjective (11/7)

Dyspnea (related to): "I feel like I can't take a deep breath"
Cough (productive): Cough with thin white sputum
Emphysema: -0- Bronchitis: -0-
Asthma: -0-
Smoker: Yes Packs/day: 1½ # of years: 15
Use of respiratory aids: -0-

Objective (11/6)

Respiratory rate: 28 regular Depth: shallow
Other: no crepitous palpated L chest/trachea midline

Breath sounds: Scattered fine crackles; rhonchi clearing some with cough; slightly diminished L lateral and both bases
Use of accessory muscles: Diaphragmatic
Nasal flaring: None
Cyanosis: Generally pale with fingernails dusky
Clubbing of fingers: -0-
Sputum characteristics: Thin, pink-tinged
Mentation/restlessness: Lethargic, arouses easily, slightly disoriented to place and time momentarily from time to time
ABGs: PO_2 89, PCO_2 38, pH 7.38

SAFETY

Subjective (11/7)

Allergies: None known per B.R. and wife (11/6); wife doesn't know what/if B.R. has taken antibiotics
History of sexually transmitted disease: -0-
Blood transfusions: None before this accident
Fractures/dislocations: None before now
Arthritis/unstable joint: -0-
Back problems: Occasional low back pain, muscle fatigue
Changes in moles: -0- Prostheses: -0-
Ambulatory devices: -0-
Vision impaired: Nearsighted Hearing impaired: -0-
Expressions of ideation of violence (self/others): -0-

Objective (11/6)

Temperature: 96.8°F rectal admission
Skin integrity: Impaired
Sores: Abrasions—abdomen/chest
Bruises: abdomen/chest. Large hematoma on L thigh; L thigh 62-cm circumference, R thigh 57-cm circumference

Scars/incisions: Midline abdomen (splenectomy 11/6)
Strength (general): Weak–pain and injuries
Muscle tone: Normal in 3 extremities, L leg deferred
ROM: R—full/L limited by fractures/pain.
Gait: Bedrest
Paresthesia: Numbness L foot Paralysis: -0-

SEXUALITY MALE:

Subjective (11/7)

Concerns/complaints: None Use of condoms: No
Penile discharge: -0- Prostate disorder: -0-
Vasectomy: -0-
Practice self-exam: Breast: No Testicles: No
Last proctoscopic exam: None
Prostate exam: With last physical several years ago

Objective (11/7)

Exam: Breast: No masses noted
Testicles: Deferred
Prostate: Deferred

SOCIAL INTERACTIONS

Subjective (11/7)

Marital status: Married/10 yr Living with: Wife and 2 children aged 4 and 7 yr
Extended family: Parents and 3 older brothers live in town
Other: Has several close friends

Role within family structure: Son/sibling/husband/father
Report of problems: -0- Coping behaviors: "Don't say much, just put up with things"
Frequency of social contacts: Frequently bowls/plays softball weekly with friends; hunts/fishes according to season

Objective (11/7)

Verbal/nonverbal communication with family/significant other(s): doesn't appear to speak much with family but acknowledges their visits with a smile or nod of head as they talk
Family interaction patterns: Wife sitting at bedside but not verbally interacting, pats his hand now and then

TEACHING/LEARNING (11/7)

Subjective

Dominant language: English
Education level: High school graduate
Learning/cognitive limitations: "I remember instructions best when I read it after I hear it"
Health beliefs/practices: "With home remedies, I'm a fast healer"
Special health-care practices: None
Familial risk factors (indicate relationship):
Cancer: -0- Heart disease: -0-
Strokes: -0- High BP: -0-
Kidney disease: -0-
Diabetes: Father (NIDDM) × 5 yr
Tuberculosis: -0- Epilepsy: -0-
Mental illness: -0-
Routine medications as stated by patient: None
Does patient take medications regularly?: N/A

Non-prescription (OTC/street) drugs: ASA occasionally, Ben-Gay

Use of alcohol (amount/frequency): Drinks beer 1 or 2 6-packs/wk

Admitting diagnosis (physician): Multiple trauma with L rib and pelvic fractures, ruptured spleen, hematoma L thigh, numerous abrasions and ecchymotic areas

Reason for hospitalization (patient): "Was in accident at work"

History of current complaint: "I was guiding a beam into place and had my head turned when all of a sudden I was pinned to the floor. I guess the beam broke free but I don't really know what happened. I broke my pelvis and some ribs. Doctor said he removed my spleen."

Other relevant illness and/or previous hospitalizations/surgeries: -0-

Evidence of failure to improve: None

Last physical exam: Several years ago

Patient expectations of this hospitalization?: "get well, be able to go back to my job"

DISCHARGE CONSIDERATIONS

Data obtained: 11/7

Anticipated discharge: 11/17

Resources: Person: wife Financial: Workmen's Compensation, some savings

Anticipated areas requiring assistance: Self-care/hygiene, transportation, ambulation (devices). Physical layout of home: Bedroom upstairs; may need to relocate on first floor initially.

CRITICAL CARE PLAN: MULTIPLE TRAUMA

PATIENT PROBLEM STATEMENT/ FOCUS (NURSING DIAGNOSIS)

Fluid volume deficit actual 2 related to vascular loss, nonfunctioning GI system evidenced by hypotension, decreased pulse volume/pressure, decreased urine output, lethargy, absence of bowel sounds.

PATIENT OUTCOMES/ EVALUATION CRITERIA

- Demonstrates improved fluid balance with skin warm, pink, and dry within 4 hours (11/6 2100).
- Urine output is greater than 40 cc/h within 4 hours (11/6 2100), revised to 10 hours (11/7 0300) accomplished,
- Vital signs within normal limits,
- Patient arousable and oriented,
- Capillary refill <3 seconds within 12 hours (11/7 0500) revised to 16 hours (11/7 0900).

Actions/Interventions	Rationale
Assess arterial and cuff blood pressure, heart rate, pulses per post-operative protocol and prn.	Cuff blood pressure/ arterial blood pressure should rise and heart rate should decrease consistent with increase in circulating blood volume.
Measure CVP q hr	Useful in evaluating replacement therapy needs. Low

Actions/Interventions	Rationale
	CVP reflects hypovolemic state due to blood/fluid loss.
Maintain integrity of invasive lines per protocol.	Provides immediate access to venous system for infusion of blood/solutions in presence of peripheral vasoconstriction. Disconnection of arterial, subclavian lines could result in exsanguination.
Measure urine hourly; record specific gravity q 4–8 hr.	Urine output of less than 35–40 cc/hr (5 ml/kg/hr) may indicate inadequate circulating volume/ decreased renal perfusion. Persistent oliguria may be indicative of renal injury. Elevated specific gravity indicates concentration of urine, which should decrease as fluid balance is restored.
Note/document color clarity of urine.	RBCs in urine may be related to kidney contusion or reduced glomerular

	filtration during hypovolemia. Myoglobin released by damaged muscle tissue can seriously damage tubules.
Assess level of consciousness; pupil response; orientation to person/place/time; response to stimuli; ability to move (Glasgow Coma Scale).	Although mental status should improve as blood volume/hemoglobin return to more normal levels, failure to improve may indicate developing complications.
Assess respiratory status:	
Rate:	Tachypnea may be associated with pain, decreased circulating volume, or respiratory compromise.
Breath sounds:	Crackles/rhonchi will likely develop because of fluid leaking into interstitial spaces (lung contusion), or could indicate fluid overload in rapid volume replacement.
Check abdominal dressings/noting	Early detection of bleeding provides

Actions/Interventions	Rationale
amount and character of drainage. Change dressings daily and prn.	opportunity to intervene appropriately.
Evaluate color and character of all secretions. Measure and hematest nasogastric contents. Hematest stools.	Early detection of stress ulcers or coagulation problems (DIC) provides opportunity for prompt intervention before excessive losses occur.
Record gastric losses q 8 hr.	Losses contribute to overall fluid status/needs and affect electrolyte balance.
Assess GI functioning noting: absence of nausea, decreased gastric secretions, presence of bowel sounds, onset of flatus/stool.	Indicates readiness to remove nasogastric tube and resume oral intake.
Observe for complaints of increased/unusual abdominal pain, sudden vomiting, increase in abdominal girth.	Signs/symptoms associated with complications: e.g., postoperative hemorrhage, mesenteric ischemic tissue pain, retroperitoneal

	hemorrhage, developing ileus, peritonitis.
Administer IV fluids:	
D5 ½ NS at 150 ml/hr	Crystalloid volume expander. Replaces sodium and fluids depleted by injury/ hemorrhage/ surgery.
Administer 1 unit packed cells now (11/6 1800). Additional unit packed red blood cells at 2400 11/6.	Restores circulating blood volume; replaces depleted components/ oxygen-carrying hemoglobin.
Monitor for transfusion reaction per protocol.	Prompt intervention may prevent serious complications/death.
Obtain Hg and Hct at 2200 11/6. Obtain CBC, plasma proteins, serum osmolality at 0600 11/7.	Evaluates effectiveness of replacement therapies and future needs.

PATIENT PROBLEM STATEMENT/ FOCUS (NURSING DIAGNOSIS)

Pain related to physical trauma, evidenced by verbal complaints, guarding of affected areas, facial grimacing, and narrowed focus.

PATIENT OUTCOMES/ EVALUATION CRITERIA

- Reports pain is minimized/controlled effective immediately and ongoing.
- Demonstrates absence of muscle tension and resting/sleeping when undisturbed within 24–48 hours (11/8 1700).
- Participates in planned activities within physical limitations within 5 days (11/11).

Actions/Interventions	Rationale
Explain activities/ procedures before beginning them.	Allows patient to prepare mentally for activity as well as participate in controlling level of discomfort.
Provide routine comfort measures: position change, back rub, Therapeutic Touch.	Pain management techniques with which patient/wife may participate.
Apply ice packs L thigh × 48 hr discontinue 1800 11/8.	Reduces edema/ hematoma formation; decreases pain sensation.
Instruct in/encourage use of relaxation exercises, deep breathing techniques.	Refocuses attention and aids patient in gaining control of situation.
Medicate before activities (e.g., deep	Provides pain relief/ muscle relaxation

breathing/coughing, repositioning).	and improves mobility/ performance.
Support injured areas during movement/ activities.	Helps prevent muscle tension/spasm to reduce associated discomfort.
Determine pain characteristics (e.g. sharp, throbbing, constant), use 1–10 scale. Accept patient's description.	Pain is subjective. Incisional pain may have different quality than pain of fractures. Use of scale provides baseline for comparison of future episodes, assesses effectiveness of analgesia, and differentiation of complications.
Monitor vital signs.	Often increased in acute pain.
Administer morphine sulfate 2–4 mg IV q 1 hr. Note/record drug effectiveness.	Morphine sulfate is usual drug of choice for severe visceral/ muscle/bone pain and is given IV because of immediate effectiveness and decreased intramuscular absorption (vasoconstriction). *Note:* Smaller IV doses can reduce

Actions/Interventions	Rationale
	side effects of respiratory depression/ hypotension.
Assess for readiness to alter/reduce drug therapy.	Progressive changes in analgesia will be required for long-term/ self-management.

PATIENT PROBLEM STATEMENT/ FOCUS (NURSING DIAGNOSIS)

Breathing Pattern, ineffective related to musculoskeletal impairment and pain, evidenced by altered chest excusion/splinting, dyspnea, tachypnea, and abnormal ABGs.

PATIENT OUTCOMES/ EVALUATION CRITERIA

- Maintains integrity of airway, and symptoms of hypoxia are absent, effective immediately/ongoing.
- Lung sounds clear, chest x-ray and ABGs normal within 72 hours (11/9 1700).

Actions/Interventions	Rationale
Maintain patent airway: correct head position, effective cough or suctioning as needed.	Breathing/ventilation may be blocked mechanically and by accumulation of secretions.

Assess respiratory status:	
Rate:	Tachypnea may be due to pain, hypovolemia, or respiratory complication such as atelectasis, ARDS or pulmonary embolus.
Chest movement (excursion):	Physiologic splinting may be present because of rib fractures/pain but changes may indicate complications, e.g., hemothorax/ pneumothorax.
Color of lips/ mucous membranes:	Pallor or cyanosis suggestive of inadequate oxygenation.
Presence of adventitious breath sounds	Crackles/rhonchi may indicate increased interstitial fluid/ edema from lung contusion, atelectasis, developing pneumonia, ARDS, or PE
Evaluate mentation.	Confusion/lethargy, etc., may indicate decreased oxygenation to brain.

Actions/Interventions	Rationale
Elevate head of bed as injuries permit.	Provides optimal lung expansion.
Encourage/assist with deep breathing/coughing exercises and use of incentive spirometer. Splint rib cage with pillow during activity.	Facilitates deeper respiratory effort, prevents/reduces atelectasis, and promotes expectoration. Provides support for fractured ribs to enhance participation.
Note character, amount, and color of sputum.	Secretions may be thick (dehydrated) and blood tinged (lung contusion). Change of sputum color/odor may indicate infection; hemoptysis (frank bleeding) signals serious complication (pulmonary infarct, DIC).
Discuss relationship of smoking to respiratory function. Assist with coping techniques during abrupt cessation of smoking.	Provides information to help patient cooperate with regimen and prevent pulmonary complications.
Assess change in character of chest discomfort,	May be indicative of developing complications

development of sudden dyspnea, tachycardia, increasing anxiety level, and/or changes in mentation.	(PE/ARDS/fat emboli) and altered gas exchange indicating need for additional laboratory evaluation (e.g., ABGs, CXR, urine for fat).
Review serial chest x-rays.	Reveals changes indicative of complications (e.g., atelectasis, ARDS, pulmonary embolus).
Review/graph ABGs.	Readily accessible information for comparison of degree of oxygenation, CO_2 retention, and need for alteration of therapy.
Administer O_2 with humidity per cannula/mask at 4 L.	Increases PO_2 and reduces ischemic muscle pain. Humidity helps mobilize secretions/prevents formation of mucous plugs.

PATIENT PROBLEM STATEMENT/ FOCUS (NURSING DIAGNOSIS)

Tissue Perfusion, altered: systemic related to hypovolemia and exchange problems evidenced by hypotension, pale/cool skin, and confusion; *peripheral:* related to decreased arterial and/or venous blood flow evidenced by diminished pulses and sensation L leg/foot.

PATIENT OUTCOMES/ EVALUATION CRITERIA

- Displays adequate systemic circulation by stable vital signs, adequate urine output, and clear mentation within 12 hours (0500, 11/7) revised to 16 hours, (0900 11/7).
- Demonstrates improved circulation to L leg by stronger pulses, pink color and increased warmth L foot and capillary refill <3 seconds L toes within 24 hours (1700 11/7).

Actions/Interventions	Rationale
Monitor vital signs, changes in mentation/level of consciousness.	Cerebral perfusion/ oxygenation is a sensitive indicator of general perfusion. Changes in mentation may also indicate presence of fat emboli.
Evaluate skin color/temperature.	Pale, clammy skin is related to compensatory mechanism during shock that shunts blood to brain and internal organs with peripheral vasoconstriction.
Measure circumference left thigh q 12 hr (0800–2000); note change from	Provides for comparison/ evaluation of increase or resolution of

baseline of L 62 cm/R 57 cm.	hematoma/tissue edema.
Assess both lower extremities noting: temperature, color, sensation, presence/quality of peripheral pulses, and capillary refill.	Impaired circulation to peripheral nerves and tissues at the time of injury may have caused temporary or permanent damage. Potential exists for increased or continuing impairment during acute phase of hematoma/edema formation. Absence or sudden reduction of pulses necessitates immediate evaluation for arterial impediment/medical intervention to prevent permanent injury.
Apply ice pack to L thigh × 48 hr (to 1800 11/8).	Reduces swelling and may help prevent further hematoma formation.
Provide passive and teach active ROM exercises for legs/feet, especially joints/digits distal to injury.	Reduces hazard of thrombophlebitis. Promotes tissue healing and joint mobility.
Monitor both lower	There is an increased

Actions/Interventions	Rationale
extremities for pain/Homan's sign.	potential for thrombophlebitis and pulmonary emboli in patients immobilized for 5 days or more.
Turn side to side with support q 2 hr. Inspect skin and bony prominences and massage as indicated.	Decreased perfusion and restricted mobility increase risk of skin breakdown.

PATIENT PROBLEM STATEMENT/ FOCUS (NURSING DIAGNOSIS)

Infection, potential for related to presence of incision, traumatized tissue; altered lung expansion and impaired ciliary action; altered peristalsis; decreased hemoglobin; and invasive procedures.

PATIENT OUTCOMES/ EVALUATION CRITERIA

- Achieves timely wound healing free of purulent drainage or erythema by 11/12.
- Demonstrates absence of nosocomial infection (ongoing).

Actions/Interventions	Rationale
Inspect incisions, dressings, and IV sites. Note/report drainage, unusual	May indicate wound infection, vein inflammation predisposing patient

pain, increased redness, and swelling.	to sepsis.
Monitor temperature q 4 hr.	Usually elevates when infection is present.
Change dressings as indicated.	Moist, bloody dressings provide medium for bacterial growth.
Investigate complaints of sudden, severe abdominal or bladder pain. Note character of urine.	Incisional infection and peritonitis can develop. Indwelling catheter provides access for bacteria, which can result in urinary tract infection.
Provide routine sterile catheter care q 8 hr prn.	Reduces risk of ascending infection.
Encourage deep breathing, incentive spirometer, exercise and reposition q 2 hr.	Mobilizes secretions and reduces/ prevents atelectasis reducing risk of pulmonary infection.
Monitor for changes in sputum characteristics.	May indicate developing respiratory tract infections.
Administer Cefotaxime IV piggyback q 4 hr.	Prevents/combats infection.

PATIENT PROBLEM STATEMENT (NURSING DIAGNOSIS) (Identified 11/7)

Anxiety, moderate related to change in health status, role functioning, threat of socioeconomic changes, evidenced by apprehension, irritability, and preoccupation with feelings of discomfort.

PATIENT OUTCOMES/ EVALUATION CRITERIA

- Appears relaxed and reports reduction of anxiety within 24 hours (0900 11/8).
- Verbalizes understanding of feelings of anxiety and demonstrates problem-solving skills within 72 hours (0900 11/10).

Actions/Interventions	Rationale
Establish therapeutic relationship: acknowledge fear and encourage B.R./wife to acknowledge and express feelings.	Provides an environment in which patient/wife can freely express feelings and begin to work on anxieties and solutions.
Give accurate information about condition/therapies.	Helps in understanding realities of the situation. It is easier to deal with reality than with fearful fantasy.
Differentiate/identify relationship of extreme anxiety to	Increased respiratory rate leads to shallower

onset of respiratory complications.

respirations, impairing oxygenation. Increased muscle tension potentiates discomfort/pain, further impairing respiratory effect. Recognition of feelings assists patient to "take control" of respiratory situation.

Provide opportunity to talk about other concerns as they arise. Let B.R. know these concerns will be listened to on an ongoing basis.

Recognizing the severity of the accident and probability of being off work for an extended period of time, will have unspoken concerns about financial/job security, family interactions/ relationships.

Refer to resources when necessary (e.g., social worker, financial advisor, counseling/therapy).

May need assistance to resolve anxiety/ deal with changes that will occur as a result of the accident.

MATERNAL PATIENT SITUATION: PRETERM LABOR/PREVENTION OF DELIVERY

Mrs. R.F.M., a 30-yr-old gravida 1, para 0, with EDD of 6/29/86, and ultrasound confirmation of two fetuses present (office visit 2/86) called physician's office today at 1400. R.F.M. had experienced a contraction beginning at 1340, and at 1400, her abdomen remained firm to touch even after she had attempted to diminish the contraction by (1) drinking two large glasses of water, (2) voiding a moderate amount, and (3) lying on her left side. She was directed to the hospital for evaluation where she was admitted with an initial diagnosis of false labor.

ADMITTING PHYSICIAN'S ORDERS

Have patient drink 480–720 cc of fluid now.
Apply external fetal monitor (EFM) and document uterine activity and fetal status.
Check cervix for dilatation and effacement.
Nitrazine test now.
Vaginal culture now.
Stat CBC, K^+, UA.
Fasting blood glucose per fingerstick in AM.
Terbutaline 0.25 mg subq and 5 mg PO now; if contractions do not cease, start 500 cc lactated Ringer's and begin terbutaline drip per protocol.
Betamethasone 12.5 mg (2 cc) IM q 12 hr × 2.
VS q 4 hr.
Complete bedrest.
Regular diet.

NURSING HISTORY AND ASSESSMENT

Name: R.F.M.
Age: 30 DOB: 5/6/55 Sex: Female
Race: Caucasian

Admission date: 3/14/86 Time: 1520
From: Home
Source of information: Patient
Father of child: R.L.M. Age: 38

ACTIVITY/REST

Subjective

Sleep: Hours: 8–10 hr/night Naps: 2/day
Aids: None
Insomnia: -0-
Usual activities/hobbies: Needlework and reading
Limitations imposed by pregnancy: Bedrest ordered by physician 2/4/86
Occupation: RN; worked parttime until 2/4/86

Objective

Observed response to activity: Cardiovascular: slight increase in rate/110
Respiratory: slight increase in rate/26
Mental status: Outgoing; alert; responds appropriately
Neuromuscular assessment:
Quality of extremities: Moves all four extremities well/equal
Posture: Erect ROM: Full Tremors: -0-
Strength: Good/equal in all extremities
Deformity: None

CIRCULATION

Subjective

History of: Elevated BP: -0-
Heart trouble: -0-
Rheumatic fever: -0- Ankle/leg edema: -0-

Phlebitis: -0- Slow healing; -0-
Extremities: Numbness: -0- Tingling: -0-
Cough/character of sputum: -0- / N/A

Objective

BP: R: Stand: 122/70
Sitting: 120/66 Lying: 120/62
L: Stand: 124/72 Sitting: 122/68
Lying: 120/62
Pulse (palpation): Peripheral—Radials 3+ Pedals 2+
Heart sounds: No murmurs or rubs
Apical rate: 100 BPM
Rhythm: Regular Quality: Strong
Jugular vein distention: -0-
Extremities: Temperature: Warm to touch
Color: Pink
Capillary refill: Rapid; less than 3 seconds
Homan's sign: -0- Varicosities: -0-
Nails: Normal; pink nailbeds; nail base, firm
Color/cyanosis: Mucous membranes: pink; intact
Conjunctiva: Salmon-colored Sclera: White

EGO INTEGRITY

Subjective

Pregnancy planned: Yes
Patient feels adjusted to pregnancy: Yes
Father feels adjusted to pregnancy: Yes
Financial concerns: None
Religion: Maternal/Paternal: Both Protestant Practicing: Yes
Cultural factors: Urban "White collar" workers, middle class
Report of stress factors: "I have had very little until

now, in the way of stress. Now I am very concerned about our babies' health."

Objective

Emotional status: Calm, fearful
Observed physiologic response(s): Remaining calm, yet demonstrates appropriate concern; facial expression tense; body tension, guarded

ELIMINATION

Subjective

Usual bowel pattern: Once a day   Laxative use: -0-
Character of stool: Soft, brown, formed
  Last BM: Yesterday
  Bleeding; -0-   Hemorrhoids: -0-
  Diarrhea: -0-   Constipation: -0-
Usual voiding pattern: Every 2–4 hr around the clock   Incontinence: -0-
  Urgency: -0-   Frequency: Since third wk of pregnancy   Retention: -0-
Character of urine: Clear, pale yellow
Pain/burning/difficulty voiding: -0-
History of kidney/bladder disease: -0-

Objective

Abdomen: slightly tender since 12/85
  Soft/firm: Firm
  Palpable mass: No abnormalities
  Size/girth: 22 cm
  Bowel sounds: Present in all four quadrants
Hemorrhoids (initial exam): None present
Bladder palpable: -0-   Overflow voiding: -0-
Urinalysis report: To be done
  Albuminuria/glycosuria: Negative per dipstick

FOOD/FLUID

Subjective

Loss of appetite: -0- Nausea: -0-
Vomiting: Severe vomiting occurred during first 15 wk of pregnancy
Mastication/swallowing problems: -0-
Heartburn/food intolerance: -0-
Normal weight: 140 lb Use of diuretics: -0-
Dietary pattern: Eats three meals/day Last ate/what: Lunch—soup and sandwich, milk, cookie

Objective

Current weight: 159 lb Height: 5′5″
Skin turgor: Good, elastic
Edema: Dependent/periorbital: -0- Jugular distention: -0-
Thyroid enlarged: No Halitosis: -0-
Condition of teeth/gums: All teeth present and in good condition/pink, no bleeding
Appearance of tongue: Pink; fully mobile within mouth
Mucous membranes: Pink; intact
Breath sounds: Clear bilateral
Hb/Hct (anemia): Hb 12.6 Hct 37.8
Diabetic screening: GTT: N/A
Thyroid studies: N/A

HYGIENE

Subjective

Activities of daily living: Independent: in all areas until 2/4/86, since then has maintained bedrest with bathroom privileges

Dependent (specify): Husband has done all household tasks since R.F.M. was placed on bedrest (2/4/86)

Objective

General appearance: Clean and neat, maternity dress, low-heeled shoes, light makeup, hair groomed
Condition of scalp: Clean, slightly dry

NEUROSENSORY

Subjective

Fainting spells/dizziness: Dizziness during first trimester
Headaches: Location: Right temporal area
Frequency: Occasional, "especially when I am under stress;" Has temporomandibular joint disease (TMJ)
Tingling/numbness (location): -0-
Seizures: -0- How controlled: N/A
Eyes/vision loss: Nearsighted R/L: corrected with glasses
Ears/hearing loss: None
Nose/epistaxis: Occasional, "especially when humidity is very low"
Sense of smell: Reports no problems/not tested

Objective

Mental status: Alert, oriented to time, person, place
Pupils: PERLA
Glasses: Yes Contacts: -0- Hearing aid: -0-
Unusual speech pattern/impairment: -0-

PAIN/COMFORT

Subjective

Location: Suprapubic Quality: Dull pain; increases when symphysis pubis is touched Duration: One week Precipitating factors: Twin "A" became engaged

How relieved: Is not relieved; tried drinking two large glasses of water and lying on left side

Objective

Facial grimacing: When area is palpated Narrowed focus: No

Guarding affected area: Asks medical staff to use light touch when taking uterine measurements

RESPIRATION

Subjective

Dyspnea/caused by: -0- Cough/productive: -0-

History: Bronchitis: -0- Asthma: -0- Tuberculosis: -0-

Smoker: -0-

Objective

Respiratory: Rate: 20/min Depth: Shallow Quality: Equal; bilateral

Breath sounds: Clear bilateral

Sputum characteristics: None at present

SAFETY

Subjective

Allergies/sensitivity: Penicillin
Reaction: Generalized red rash occurred when patient was a child, has not taken penicillin since
History of STD (date/type): -0-
German measles: Immune
Exposure to radiation: Not during pregnancy
Previous obstetric problems: N/A
ABO/Rh sensitivity: N/A
Blood transfusion: -0-
Fractures/dislocations: Nose was fractured at age 4
Arthritis/unstable joints: -0-   Back problems: -0-
Changes in moles: -0-   Enlarged nodes: -0-
Impaired: Vision: Wears glasses   Hearing: -0-
Prosthesis: -0-   Ambulatory devices: -0-

Objective

Temperature: 98.6°F PO
Skin integrity: intact   Rashes: -0-   Sores: -0-
Bruises: -0-
Scars: Inner right forearm, old injury from childhood
Strength (general): Good; equal in all four extremities
Muscle tone: Firm   Gait: Normal
ROM: Good
Paresthesia/paralysis: -0-
Fetal: Heart rate: Twin "A" 150 BPM; Twin "B" 154 BPM
Location: Twin "A": LLQ (2 fingers above pubic bone); Twin "B": URQ (four fingers breadth to R of umbilicus)
Method of auscultation: EFM
Fundal height: 22 cm
Estimated gestation: 24 1/7th wk

Movement: Frequent; active
Ballottement: Absent; Twin "A": engaged
Blood Type/Rh: Maternal: A+ Paternal: A+
Screens: Sickle cell: N/A Rubella: Immune
Hepatitis: -0- AFP: -0-
Serology syphilis: Negative
Cervical/rectal culture: Pending (done 3/14/86; 1600)
Vaginal warts/lesions: -0-

SEXUALITY FEMALE:

Subjective

Menarche: 10 years old Length of cycle: 28 days Duration: 3–5 days
Last menstrual period (LMP): 9/19/85 Amount: Moderate EDD: 6/29/86
Vaginal discharge: Odorless, clear, thick
Bleeding since LMP: Once a month, first trimester spotting
Practices breast self-exam: Yes
Last PAP smear: 11/19/85 Recent contraceptive method: Diaphragm
OB history: Gravida: 1 Para: 0 Abortions: 0 Now living: 0 Full term: 0 Premature: 0 Multiple births: 0

Objective

Pelvic: Vulva: Pink; moist Perineum: No abnormalities; pink; intact
Vagina: Dark, pink Cervix: Closed; Chadwick's sign present
Uterus: Distended, pear-shaped
Adnexal: Normal

Diagonal conjugate: 12.5 cm   Transverse diameter: Outlet: 10.5 cm
Shape of sacrum: Normal, average inclination-
Coccyx: Movable
Ischial spines: >8 cm
Inlet: Adequate   Mid: Adequate
Outlet: Adequate
Prognosis for delivery: Good for vaginal delivery
Breast exam: Supple, symmetric; no abnormalities
Nipples: erect/dark in color; no cracks or fissures; no abnormalities
Serology test: Negative 10/25/85

SOCIAL INTERACTIONS

Subjective

Relationship status: Married   Years in relationship: 8
Living with: Husband
Role within family structure: Housewife; secondary breadwinner
Extended family: Married younger brother/nephew in town, all other relatives live out of town
Other support person(s): Many close friends in town; mother available to come if patient goes home on bedrest
Report of problems: -0-

Objective

Verbal/nonverbal communication with family/significant other(s): Husband sitting beside bed, speaks quietly and holds patient's hand

TEACHING/LEARNING

Subjective

Language dominant: English
Education: R.F.M., bachelor's degree

Husband: Master's degree Occupation: Respiratory therapist

Familial risk factors (maternal/paternal: indicate relationship)

Tuberculosis: Maternal grandfather Diabetes: -0- High BP: Maternal aunt

Epilepsy: -0- Heart disease: -0-

Strokes: -0- Kidney disease: -0-

Cancer: maternal grandmother Multiple births: maternal side: Aunt had twins; father of these babies is a twin Genetic problems: -0-

Prescribed medications: Drug: Maternal prenatal vitamin/mineral supplement: Dose one tablet daily

Schedule: 2200 every day

Take regularly: Yes

Nonprescription drugs: OTC: -0- Illicit: -0-

Use of alcohol (amount/frequency): -0-

Current complaints/symptoms of pregnancy: Called OB at 1400, C/O "having a contraction that didn't seem to go away" and abdomen remained very firm

Relevant illnesses and/or hospitalization/surgery: 12/10/85: short stay hospitalization for IV therapy; R.F.M. experienced 7-lb weight loss in 48 hr due to severe prenatal vomiting

Last physical exam: Last OB appointment, 3/7/86; uterine measurement, FHT, and ultrasound done by: Dr. R.P. Ultrasound report: Twin "A" was shown to be engaged, and both babies were growing at the same rate. R.F.M. complained of frequent regular contractions and the day after the appointment called to report loss of mucus plug.

Expectations of this pregnancy: Full-term, healthy babies

Type of delivery planned: Vaginal, although twin "B" is breech so realizes a possibility of a C-section is present

Type of anesthesia planned: Local, if episiotomy is done; otherwise, none
Type of infant feeding planned: Breast

Preparation: Prenatal/intrapartal
Classes: Prematurity Prevention 2/18/86 Infant care/feeding: No formal class yet; was to begin childbirth classes 3/31/86.
Books: Several medical books dealing with obstetrics and bonding
Other (specify): Contacted the local chapters of La Leche League and the Twins Club

DISCHARGE PLAN CONSIDERATIONS

If delivery delayed: Will require periodic home health monitoring/visitation; homemaker assistance

Anticipated discharge: Within 7–10 days.

Resources available: Husband, mother

MATERNAL CARE PLAN: PRETERM LABOR/PREVENTION OF DELIVERY

PATIENT PROBLEM STATEMENT/ FOCUS (NURSING DIAGNOSIS)

Anxiety moderate related to the possibility of premature delivery, perceived or actual threat to fetuses and self-evidenced by expressions of concern regarding current events, increased tension, apprehension, and narrowed focus.

PATIENT OUTCOMES/ EVALUATION CRITERIA

- Verbalizes awareness of feelings of anxiety within 24 hours (1600 3/15).
- Appears relaxed and reports anxiety is reduced to a manageable level within 24 hours (1600 3/15).
- Identifies three ways she is dealing with anxieties within 48 hours (1600 3/16).

Actions/Interventions	Rationale
Introduce self to R.F.M./family. Maintain "primary caregiver."	Important for patient/husband to feel "connected" to the caregiver to promote a sense of trust.
Explain procedures, nursing interventions, and treatments.	Knowledge of the reasons for these activities can decrease fear of the unknown.

Orient R.F.M. and husband to labor suite environment.	Helps patient/husband to feel at ease and more comfortable in their surroundings.
Keep communication open; discuss the possible side effects and outcomes, maintaining an optimistic attitude.	Knowing information will be given freely and questions will be answered can help to reduce anxiety and promote hope and strengthen "working" relationship between patient and staff.
Control external stimulation. Review restrictions/ rationale (e.g., TV, radio, visitors, phone).	Quiet atmosphere promotes rest and relaxation, which can assist in decreasing uterine activity and perceived or actual threat to fetuses.
Encourage use of relaxation techniques (e.g., deep breathing exercises, visualization, guided imagery).	Enables the patient to obtain maximal benefit from rest periods; prevents muscle fatigue and may improve uterine blood flow. Provides opportunity for active participation and enhances sense of control.
Encourage	Helps patient to

Actions/Interventions	Rationale
verbalization of fears and concerns.	define and become aware of specific problems, providing opportunity for problem solving and thereby reducing anxiety.
Monitor maternal/fetal vital signs as indicated.	Vital signs of patient and fetuses may be altered by anxiety. Stabilization may reflect reduction of anxiety level.
Assess support systems available to R.F.M./couple.	Availability of the assistance and caring of significant others, including caregivers, is extremely important during this time of stress and uncertainty to decrease anxiety and enhance coping.

PATIENT PROBLEM STATEMENT/ FOCUS (NURSING DIAGNOSIS)

Activity intolerance related to muscle/cellular hypersensitivity evidenced by increased uterine irritability and cervical dilatation; and adverse effect on uteroplacental perfusion evidenced by change in fetal heart rate.

PATIENT OUTCOMES/ EVALUATION CRITERIA

- Reports/displays cessation of uterine contractions within 12–36 hours (0400 3/14–15).

Actions/Interventions	Rationale
Expedite the admissions process and institute bedrest using left lateral position.	Facilitating reduction of activity/ psychologic stressors may help uterine contractions to cease. Left-lateral position improves uterine flow and may decrease uterine irritability.
Explain the reasons for requiring bedrest, lying on left side, and decreasing activity.	These measures are intended to keep the pressure of the fetus off the cervix and to enhance placental perfusion. Bedrest may decrease uterine irritability.
Demonstrate/ encourage use of relaxation techniques.	Helps reduce muscle tension and patient's perception of discomfort.
Provide nursing comfort measures such as changes of position/linen, back rub, and Therapeutic Touch.	Relieves muscle fatigue and promotes sense of well-being.

Actions/Interventions	Rationale
Decrease stimuli in room (e.g., lighting).	
Offer diversional activities, such as reading, television, or visits with selected friends or family as appropriate.	Refocuses attention, reduces boredom, and may enhance coping ability.
Monitor maternal and fetal vital signs.	Reflects effectiveness of interventions.

PATIENT PROBLEM STATEMENT/ FOCUS (NURSING DIAGNOSIS)

Poisoning, potential for related to possibility of toxic side effects (cardiovascular) of treatments and medications used to stop labor.

PATIENT OUTCOMES/ EVALUATION CRITERIA

- Verbalizes understanding of potential dangers, maternal/fetal side effects within 4 hours (2000 3/14).
- Displays no untoward effects/complications (ongoing).

Actions/Interventions	Rationale
Place R.F.M. in left-lateral position. Elevate head of bed slightly.	Decreases uterine irritability, increases placental perfusion, and

prevents supine hypotension.

Have R.F.M. drink 480–720 cc of fluid now.

To rule out preterm labor related to dehydration.

Assist as needed with sterile vaginal examination. Obtain vaginal culture on admission.

Necessary to assess cervical status, however, vaginal examinations are kept to a minimum because they may contribute to uterine irritability. Safety of tocolytic agents when cervix is greater than 4 cm dilated or 80 percent effaced is not documented. Culture is done to rule out infection and sexually transmitted diseases.

Apply external fetal monitor and assess uterine contractions and fetal heart rate electronically on admission and continuously until stable, then bid (0900, 2000).

Tactile and electronic monitoring of uterine contractions and fetal heart rate provides ongoing fetal/uterine assessment and basis for altering or maintaining drug administration. *Note:* External monitors may increase contractions in some patients.

Actions/Interventions	Rationale
Provide information about the actions and side effects of drug therapy. Obtain permit for administration of terbutaline sulfate.	Important for the patient/couple to know the purpose of the drug(s) being administered. Terbutaline sulfate is still considered an experimental drug and may cause fetal tachycardia, hyperglycemia, acidosis, and hypoxia.
Administer Terbutaline 0.25 mg subq and 5 mg PO now. Document response.	Promotes relaxation of uterine muscle and vessel walls.
Monitor vital signs q 4 hr, noting cardiac rhythm. Auscultate lung sounds. Record intake and output.	Terbutaline sulfate, which stimulates type II beta receptors, may cause complications such as cardiac tachycardia/dysrhythmias and an increase in plasma volume.
Observe for development of side effects (e.g., palpitations, increased respiratory rate, chest pain, dyspnea,	Prompt action can reverse untoward/toxic effects.

agitation). If present: discontinue drug, give oxygen per mask, start lactated Ringer's (fluid expander), administer mild sedation (Seconal 100 mg, Dalmane 15 mg, or Vistaril 25 mg) per protocol, and notify physician.	
Maintain fluid intake between 2000 and 3000 ml per day.	Amniotic fluid exchange occurs every 3–4 hours so it is advisable to have a drink every two hours and maintain high daily fluid intake.
Weigh patient daily.	Detects fluid shifts/retention, possible alteration in urinary functioning, and adequacy of nutritional intake.
Obtain urine sample for routine urinalysis.	Urinary tract infection may cause/enhance uterine irritability.
Review/monitor laboratory findings (i.e., CBC; UA; cultures; serum glucose, and potassium).	Check for anemia and presence of infection. Terbutaline sulfate causes movement of potassium ions into cells, decreasing

Actions/Interventions	Rationale
	plasma levels, increasing blood glucose and plasma insulin levels, and stimulating release of glycogen from muscle and liver.

PATIENT PROBLEM STATEMENT/ FOCUS (NURSING DIAGNOSIS)

Injury, potential for, fetal related to insufficient development to maintain physiologic self outside of uterine environment if delivered prematurely.

PATIENT OUTCOMES/ EVALUATION CRITERIA

- Maintains pregnancy until fetal viability is reached (at least 25 weeks, longer if possible).

Actions/Interventions	Rationale
Do nitrazine test now.	Verifies ruptured membranes (PROM), which presents increased risk of infection and affects choice of interventions/timing of delivery.
Assess for maternal conditions that would contraindicate	In PIH and chorioamnionitis, steroid therapy may aggravate

steroid therapy.	hypertension and mask signs of infection. Steroids may increase blood glucose levels in the patient with diabetes.
Assess fetal heart rate; note presence of uterine activity or cervical dilation.	Tocolytics can increase fetal heart rate. Delivery may be extremely rapid with small infant if persistent uterine contractions are unresponsive to tocolytics or if cervical changes continue.
Review advantages and disadvantages of steroid therapy with patient/couple.	Steroid therapy is most effective between 28 and 34 weeks gestation to stimulate lung maturity. Long-term effects on the development of the child cannot be known until longitudinal studies have been completed.
Administer betamethasone 12.5 mg (2 cc) IM q 12 hr × 2 (1800, 0600).	Although steroid therapy is still controversial, research indicates that it prevents or decreases the severity of

Actions/Interventions	Rationale
	respiratory distress syndrome by stimulating fetal surfactant production.
Stress necessity of follow-up care if discharged without delivering.	If fetuses are not delivered within 7 days of administration of steroids, dose should be repeated weekly.

PATIENT PROBLEM STATEMENT/ FOCUS (NURSING DIAGNOSIS)

Knowledge deficit [learning need] preterm labor related to lack of information/misinterpretation evidenced by questions and expression of concerns.

PATIENT OUTCOMES/ EVALUATION CRITERIA

- Verbalizes awareness of implications and possible outcomes of preterm labor within 16 hours (0800 3/15).
- Asks questions appropriately and assumes responsibility for own learning and participates in learning process within 48 hours of admission (1600 3/16).

Actions/Interventions	Rationale
Ascertain R.F.M.'s knowledge about	Establishes data base and identifies

preterm labor and possible outcomes.	individual patient learning needs.
Assess readiness to learn.	Factors such as anxiety or lack of awareness of need for information (denial) can interfere with readiness to learn.
Include husband in the teaching process.	Support from significant other(s) can help allay anxiety as well as reinforce learning.
Review signs and symptoms of "early" labor.	Helps patient to recognize preterm labor so that therapy to suppress this labor can be initiated or reinstituted promptly.
Discuss need for bedrest, limitation of activity, and restriction of sexual and nipple activity.	Activity, orgasm, and stimulation of the nipples (which releases oxytocin) may stimulate uterine activity.
Stress avoidance of use of over-the-counter (OTC) drugs while tocolytic agents are administered unless approved by physician.	Concurrent use of OTC drugs may cause deleterious effects, especially if drug has similar side effects of tocolytic agent (e.g., antihistamines or

Actions/Interventions	Rationale
	inhalers with bronchodilating effects, such as Primatene Mist).
Recommend taking oral tocolytic agents with food if drug is continued.	Food improves tolerance to drug and reduces GI side effects.
Provide information about follow-up care.	Cooperation is enhanced when patient understands need/necessity of regular monitoring/ treatment.
Arrange for visit to neonatal intensive care unit.	Helps alleviate fears and facilitates adjustment to the potential realities of the situation.
Refer to community health nurse, childbirth education class, Parents of Twins group, or another couple who have experienced a similar episode with a successful outcome.	Additional help may assist patient/couple to cope with situation, especially if she returns home to await delivery.

PSYCHIATRIC PATIENT SITUATION: ANOREXIA NERVOSA/BULIMIA

M.J.B., a 33-year-old woman, presented at her doctor's office with complaints of lightheadedness, fatigue, weakness, and a history of eating disorders. She was admitted to the Eating Disorders program on referral by her family physician for controlled environment and monitoring of physiologic well-being.

ADMITTING PHYSICIAN'S ORDERS

CBC, electrolytes, blood sugar on admission.
Endocrine studies, dexamethasone suppression test (DST) in AM.
Urinalysis in AM.
ECG in AM.
Regular diet with selective menu, schedule dietary consult.
Weigh on admission and according to protocol.
Trilafon 8 mg/tid.

NURSING HISTORY and ASSESSMENT

Name: M.J.B.
Age: 33 DOB: 2/13/54 Sex: Female
Race: Caucasian
Admission date: 6/23/87 Time: 3:30 PM
From: Home
Source of information: Self
Reliability (scale 1–4): 2 to 3 (inconsistencies in data presented)
Family member/significant other(s): Family not in area, no contact. Friend: Mrs. C.P.

ACTIVITY/REST

Subjective

Occupation: Receptionist, city government office
Usual activities/hobbies: Volunteers for church, says has "lots of projects, but can't get them completed," "would like to learn new vocation"
Leisure–time activities: "Not much. I don't like to get out with people, and I just don't seem to have the energy"
Limitations imposed by condition: "Afraid people will know about my problem"
Sleep: "Not enough, maybe 4–5 hours"
Insomnia: "I have some problem, usually because I don't get to bed." Says this is her "binge time," finds things to do to avoid going to bed.
Not rested on awakening, "tired all the time"

Objective

Observed response to activity:
Respiratory: tachypnea/28
Cardiovascular: elevated pulse/110
Mental status: Withdrawn
Posture: Sits hunched over, not looking up

CIRCULATION

Subjective

History of: Occasional ankle/leg edema

Objective

BP: 106/68 lying 90/63 sitting Pulse: 104 at rest
Heart sounds/breath sounds: Deferred

Color: Skin pale Conjunctiva/mucous membranes/ lips: Pale

EGO INTEGRITY

Subjective

What kind of person are you: "I'm a nothing, a zero"
What do you think of your body: "I don't like my body, it's too fat."
Doesn't do anything where she has to expose her body. Would like to learn massage, but doesn't want to have a man touch her body (a requirement of the class is that students practice on one another).
How would you rate your self-esteem (scale 1–10): "Zero"
What are your moods: "Depressed, lonely"
Are you a nervous person: "Yes"
Are your feelings easily hurt: "Yes. I'm afraid I'm a bother to other people. They think I'm not doing a good job. I can tell by the way they look at me."
Report of stress factors: Worries about "everything", binge eating, having to deal with people in her job, limited income, no savings or health insurance.
Previous patterns of coping with stress: Has been anorectic in the past, avoided eating, ran (frequently 10 miles a day); withdrawal (ran away from the hospital last time she was hospitalized)
Financial concerns: Is in a low-paying job, no resources
Relationship status: Single, has never been married nor had a relationship. Says "I don't like men. I can't trust them"
Cultural factors: White, middle class.
Lifestyle: Has no home of her own, house-sits for people who are gone, stays with church friends

between house-sitting jobs ("helps with the money"). Is alone a lot in this situation

Significant losses/changes (date): Left home and moved to another state 10 years ago. Does not have contact with family (family does not know where she is). Father died 4 years ago; did not see him or return for funeral

Stage of grief/manifestations of loss: Stated matter-of-factly, "I don't want to have any contact with family. I was glad to get away from them and really don't want to have any contact with them now."

Religion: Practicing Catholic, attends church several times/week

Objective

Emotional status: Calm, cooperative, fearful, anxious, dependent.

Behavior: Consistent. Verbal responses are congruent. Speech is modulated, congruent; voice low

Defense mechanisms: Uses rationalization—"I ate lunch, some lettuce and sunflower seeds;" denial —"I'm not a worthwhile person;" and projection —"I don't like the way people act, they lie, cheat and steal."

Body language: Sitting quietly with head down, looks up occasionally, and maintains eye contact when she does; "nervously twisting" tissue

ELIMINATION

Subjective

Usual bowel pattern: Irregular, constipation an ongoing problem

Uses an herbal laxative once or twice a week. Last BM: 2 days ago
Character: Dry, light-colored
Usual voiding pattern: No problem but voids infrequently (once/twice a day)
Character of urine: Dark yellow

Objective

Deferred

FOOD/FLUID

Subjective

Usual diet: Vegetarian and does not eat eggs or chicken. Eats one meal a day; no breakfast; snacks on lettuce, nuts, may have tuna for lunch. "Afraid to eat for fear I can't stop." Binges on whatever is available, usually carbohydrates (candy bars, cookies). Drinks occasional glass of water, diet colas (2–3/day).
Usual weight: 130 lb; no recent weight changes. Weighed 85 lb when she was hospitalized for anorexia the first time, 12 years ago. Vomiting: "Usually once a day, sometimes only two or three times a week"
Swallowing problem: Sore mouth and throat frequently

Objective

Current weight: 128 lb Height: 5′4″
Body build: Slight Skin turgor: Tight
Mucous membranes/lips: Dry Edema: -0-
Condition of teeth/gums: Tooth decay/erosion evident, gums inflamed, salivary glands slightly swollen. Halitosis: Sour breath

HYGIENE

Subjective

Independent in self-care

Objective

General appearance: Neatly dressed in boxy style blue suit; oxford type shoes, in good condition; dark, short hair curled around face; eye makeup lightly applied; nails well-kept, no nail polish; no jewelry noted.

NEUROSENSORY

Subjective

Sees self as "fat" even though others don't
Fainting spells/dizziness: Several times a week
Recurrent headaches: Tires easily but believes she works hard
Eyes: No complaints of eye strain or change in acuity. Does not wear glasses.
Hearing: No problems
Says concerned because she is not remembering things, "being forgetful"
States she is "depressed, feels tense and anxious, empty"

Objective

Mental status: Alert and oriented to time, place and person. Memory of immediate, recent, and remote incidents intact.

Intellectual functioning: States she has a problem concentrating and difficulty making decisions

Thought processes: Speech pattern is normal. Thinking seems fairly rational and logical with organized, coherent flow of ideas. Occasional evidence of distorted thinking (e.g., "I'm afraid my electrolytes are out of balance, but I take vitamins every day"). Speaks in a quiet voice. Defensive thinking is apparent with occasional ideas of reference: "people will say I'm weird if they find out about me"

Mood: Depressed, fearful, consistent, verbalizes feelings appropriate to the situation

Affect: Behavior is consistent with expression of feelings

Insight: Demonstrates some awareness of extent of condition. Says "I think my electrolytes are out of balance." Verbalizes awareness of not being sure she wants to give up behavior. "What will I have if I don't binge/purge anymore?" States "it makes her feel, knows she is alive."

PAIN/COMFORT

Subjective

No complaints of pain at present

Headaches occasionally "all over head", 2–3 times/wk last 3 months

Says did not have headaches until recently when vomiting became more frequent.

RESPIRATION

Subjective

Dyspnea with exertion

Does not smoke. Says does not cough except with colds.

Objective

Respiratory rate: 28 with activity/22 at rest

SAFETY

Subjective

Temperature: 99.4°F PO
No history of accidents/injuries
No known allergies
States has frequent colds, "every few months"
Expressions of ideation of violence (self/others): Says she has thoughts of "being better off dead" occasionally but would not act on them, recognizes bulimic behavior as suicidal

Objective

Nothing significant

SEXUALITY FEMALE:

Subjective

Age at menarche: 12 yr Length of cycle: Irregular Duration: 2 days
Last menstrual period: 2 months ago
Is not sexually involved with anyone and does not use birth control
Sexual abuse/incest: No

Objective

Deferred

SOCIAL INTERACTIONS

Subjective

Memory of early years: Father—alcoholic; mother—rejecting person who often told the children she wished she had not gotten married or had children. Physical abuse common in the family. Reports father occasionally "belted" mother; children were frequently "beaten" when they had displeased parents/done something wrong.

Marital status: Single. Living with church friends, house-sitting.

Genogram: Deferred to 6/24/87

Family dynamics: "Mother was angry with father most of the time." Sister and brother are 2 and 5 years younger, says "felt responsible for them when they were little, grew apart as I became older." Has not had contact with them in past 10 years.

Extended family: None

Other support persons: Employer; church friends, including Mr. and Mrs. C.P., an older couple whom she describes as surrogate parents

Role within family structure: Oldest child with younger sister and brother

Report of problems: Says feels lonely, doesn't have friends, knows she has to stop the bingeing/vomiting cycle. Doesn't trust people. Does have limited relationship with church friends, doesn't want them to know about her problem.

Coping behaviors: Preoccupation with food and compulsive need to binge/purge, withdrawal from interaction with others

Frequency of social contacts (other than work): None other than church; attends mass once or twice a week

Objective

Has not been observed with significant other(s)

TEACHING/LEARNING

Subjective

Dominant language: English
Education level: High school; graduated from secretarial/business program
Learning disabilities/cognitive limitations: Not aware of any
Health beliefs/practices: Vegetarian. Believes if she eats something, she "cannot" stop. Believes if she eats sugar, her body craves it and she will just keep on eating.
Familial risk factors: Father died of stroke, age 67, maternal grandmother had a "bad" heart. Not aware of any other significant family history, although mother was "not well (PMS?)."
Prescribed medications: None
Non-prescription drugs: Does not take any OTC or illicit drugs. Takes an herbal laxative once or twice a week. Takes vitamins "because I know I don't eat right."
Use of alcohol: None
Admitting diagnosis (physician): anorexia/bulimia DSM III-R Axis 307.10
Reason for hospitalization (patient): "to get my electrolytes under control"
History of current complaint: long-standing eating problems (20 yr), anorexic as an adolescent, bingeing and purging for last 10 years.
Patient expectations of this hospitalization: "I want to begin to feel good about myself and my work, spiritually, mentally, and physically"
Previous hospitalization: Hospitalized twice 10 and 12 years ago. Ran away from the hospital the last time and moved to another state.
Evidence of failure to improve: Physical: Having blackouts, fainting spells, says "electrolytes are out of balance." Mental: States has difficulty

thinking, relaxing; complains of inferiority feelings.
Date of last physical exam: Fall 1983

DISCHARGE PLAN CONSIDERATIONS

Date data obtained: 6/23
Anticipated date of discharge: 7/14 (21 days)
Resources available: Persons: Employer and church friends.
Financial: Has job "not doing what she was trained to do," which employer will hold for her. Has no insurance or savings.
Anticipated changes in living after discharge: None, at the moment. Would like to get own place as soon as feasible.
Living facility other than home: Would like to continue to house-sit, "helps with the money"
Community supports: Church Socialization: No social activities

PSYCHIATRIC CARE PLAN: ANOREXIA NERVOSA/BULIMIA

PATIENT PROBLEM STATEMENT/ FOCUS (NURSING DIAGNOSIS)

Nutrition, altered: less than body requirements related to inadequate food intake and self-induced vomiting evidenced by pale conjunctiva and mucous membranes, poor skin turgor, inflamed gums, tooth decay/erosion, slightly swollen salivary glands, and complaints of sore mouth/throat.

PATIENT OUTCOMES/ EVALUATION CRITERIA

Short-term

• Verbalizes understanding of nutritional needs within 72 hours (3 PM 6/26).

• Establishes a dietary pattern with caloric intake adequate to maintain appropriate weight within 72 hours (3 PM 6/26).

• Abstains from bingeing or vomiting for duration of the program.

Intermediate/long-term:

• Displays stable weight at 3- and 6-month intervals.

• Reports continued abstinence from binge/purge episodes (ongoing).

Actions/Interventions	Rationale
Establish a minimum weight goal to be maintained: 125–130 lb.	When this is agreed upon, psychologic work can begin. Malnutrition is a mood-altering condition leading to depression and agitation so that

	adequate nutrition is important for psychologic well-being.
Maintain a regular weighing schedule, Monday–Wednesday–Friday, before breakfast in same attire and graph results.	Provides accurate ongoing record of weight loss and/or gain. Also diminishes obsessing about gains and/or losses.
Make selective menu available and allow M.J.B. to control choices.	Patient needs to gain confidence in self and feel in control of environment. More likely to eat preferred foods.
Be alert to choices of low calorie foods, hoarding food, and disposing of food in various places such as pockets or wastebaskets.	Patient may try to avoid taking in what she views as excessive calories.
Use a consistent approach. Present and remove food without persuasion and/or comment. Sit with M.J.B. while eating, also without comment.	Patient detects urgency and reacts to pressure. When staff respond in a consistent manner, patient can begin to trust her responses. Avoids manipulative games. Any comment that might be seen as coercion

Actions/Interventions	Rationale
	provides focus on food. Patient may experience guilt if forced to eat. The one area in which she has exercised power and control is food/eating. Structuring meals and decreasing discussions about food will decrease power struggles with patient.
Provide one-to-one supervision. Have M.J.B. remain in the room with no bathroom privileges for a specified period (½ hr) following eating.	Prevents vomiting during/after eating. *Note:* Sometimes patients desire food and use a binge–purge syndrome to maintain weight. Purging may occur for the first time in a patient as a response to establishment of weight program.
Avoid room checks and control devices.	Reinforces feelings of powerlessness and are usually not helpful because external control does not help to establish patient's own internal control.

Establish exercise program with M.J.B., discussing likes and dislikes (e.g., walking, aerobics, swimming).	A gradually increasing exercise program can help patient begin to improve muscle tone and control weight in a more satisfactory manner.
Monitor exercise program and set limits on physical activities. Chart activity/level of work (pacing, etc.).	Patient may exercise excessively to burn calories/compensate for increased intake. *Note:* Strenuous exercise may put added stress on the heart.
Provide regular diet and snacks with substitutes and preferred foods available.	Having a variety of foods available will enable patient to have a choice of potentially enjoyable foods and may enhance intake.
Carry out program of behavior modification. Involve M.J.B. in setting up program. Provide reward for maintaining weight, ignore gain/loss.	Provides structured eating situation while allowing patient some control in choices. *Note:* Behavior modification may be effective only in mild cases or for short-term weight maintenance.
Avoid giving laxatives.	Use is counterproductive as they may be used by patient to

Actions/Interventions	Rationale
	rid body of food/calories.
Schedule dietary consultation.	Helpful in establishing individual dietary needs/program and provides educational opportunity.
Administer perphenazine (Trilafon) 8 mg tid (0800, 1400, and 2200).	Antipsychotic drug that blocks postsynaptic dopamine receptors in the brain. Given to manage underlying pathology (e.g., depression/anxiety).
Review laboratory studies (i.e., blood sugar, CBC, endocrine studies).	Provides information about dietary status/needs/ effectiveness of therapy.

PATIENT PROBLEM STATEMENT/ FOCUS (NURSING DIAGNOSIS)

Fluid Volume, deficit, actual 2 related to inadequate intake of food/liquids and consistent self-induced vomiting evidenced by dry skin/mucous membranes, decreased skin turgor, altered vital signs (heart rate 104, temperature 99.4°F, orthostatic drop in BP of 16 points systolic), concentrated urine/decreased urine output, and change in mental state/memory.

PATIENT OUTCOMES/ EVALUATION CRITERIA

Short-term:

• Reports fluid intake of 2000 cc/day with increased urine output within 39 hours (6 AM 6/25).

• Demonstrates improvement in vital signs, skins turgor, and moisture of mucous membranes within three days (6/26).

• Verbalizes understanding of causative factors and behaviors necessary to correct fluid deficit within 7 days (6/30).

Long-term:

• Maintains above parameters at 3–6 month check.

Actions/Interventions	Rationale
Discuss strategies to stop vomiting (e.g., saying positive affirmation of "I can stop vomiting," talking to friend/therapist, use of imagery/relaxation).	Helping the patient to deal with feelings of anxiety, which lead to vomiting and making a decision to stop will prevent continued fluid loss.
Have M.J.B. measure urine output accurately times 3 days (6/24–26) and periodically as indicated.	Reduced urinary output may be a direct result of reduced food/fluid intake and continued vomiting.
Monitor amount and types of fluid intake. Be aware of diet soft-drink and caffeine intake.	Patient may abstain from all intake or substitute fluids for calorie intake, impacting fluid balance/renal function. Increased intake of diet soft

Actions/Interventions	Rationale
	drinks results in adequate output, even though there is no protein/calorie intake.
Monitor vital signs, capillary refill, and dizziness. Recommend rising slowly, sitting, then standing.	Orthostatic hypotension can occur with fluid deficit.
Note complaints of muscle pain/cramps, generalized weakness, paresthesia, nausea.	These are signs of potassium deficit and may reflect inadequate intake, starvation state, or deficit from self-induced vomiting.
Discuss actions necessary to regain optimal fluid balance (e.g., drinking a glass of fluid every 2 hours). Encourage use of calorie-containing beverages as well as water.	Involving patient in plan to correct fluid imbalances may enhance success and provides sense of control over what is happening to her.
Review laboratory studies (i.e., electrolytes, CBC, urinalysis).	Syndrome may result in electrolyte imbalances and hemoconcentration.

PATIENT PROBLEM STATEMENT/ FOCUS (NURSING DIAGNOSIS)

Thought processes, altered related to severe malnutrition, psychologic conflicts (e.g., sense of low self-worth, perceived lack of control), evidenced by impaired ability to make decisions, problem solve, non-reality-based verbalizations (e.g., "I need to lose 30 lb," "I ate a lot of food today, sesame seeds and lettuce"), ideas of reference (says people think she isn't doing a good job), altered sleep patterns (goes to bed after midnight, often 2 AM, gets up early), and altered attention span—distractibility.

PATIENT OUTCOMES/ EVALUATION CRITERIA

Short-term:

- Verbalizes awareness and understanding of relationship of lack of food intake to problems of concentration and decision making within 24 hours (3 PM 6/24).

Intermediate/long-term:

- Demonstrates improved ability to make decisions, problem solve, and memory of daily/ recent events within 3 weeks (7/13) with continuation at 3 to 6 month check.

Actions/Interventions	Rationale
Be aware of M.J.B.'s distorted thinking ability.	Allows the caregiver to lower expectations and provide information and support.
Listen to and do not challenge irrational, illogical thinking. Present reality	It is not possible to respond logically when thinking ability is

Actions/Interventions	Rationale
concisely and briefly.	physiologically impaired. The patient needs to hear reality, but challenging may lead to distrust and frustration.
Encourage strict adherence to nutritional regimen.	Improved nutrition is essential to improved brain functioning. (Refer to Nursing Diagnosis: Nutrition, alteration in, less than body requirements.)

PATIENT PROBLEM STATEMENT/ FOCUS (NURSING DIAGNOSIS)

Self-esteem/Body Image disturbance related to morbid fear of obesity; perceived loss of control in some aspect of life (e.g., ability to interact satisfactorily with others, eating); unmet dependency needs evidenced by distorted body image, view of self as fat, even in the presence of normal body weight (states "need to lose 30 lb"); and feels "powerless to prevent binge/purging and make changes in my life"; perceptual disturbances with failure to recognize hunger; presence of fatigue, anxiety, and depression.

PATIENT OUTCOMES/ EVALUATION CRITERIA

Short-term:
- Identifies physical assets/strengths (beginning day 1 and ongoing).

Intermediate:
- Acknowledges self as an individual who has responsibility for own actions and voluntarily stops bingeing and purging by the end of the program (3 weeks).

Long-term:
- Accepts compliments and verbalizes a more realistic body image within 3 months.

Actions/Interventions	Rationale
Establish a therapeutic nurse/ patient relationship.	Within a helping relationship, the patient can begin to trust and try out new thinking and behaviors.
Promote self-concept without moral judgement.	Patient sees herself as weak-willed, even though a part of her may feel a sense of power and control.
State rules regarding: weighing schedule, remaining in sight during medication and eating times, and consequences of not following the rules. Be consistent in carrying out rules without undue comment.	Patient is obsessed with fear of weight gain. Regular monitoring of patient's weight is important to nutritional status. Consistency is important in establishing trust. As part of the

Actions/Interventions	Rationale
	behavior modification program, the patient knows the risks involved in not following established rules (e.g., a decrease in privileges). Failure to follow rules is viewed as the patient's choice and accepted by the staff in matter-of-fact manner so as not to provide reinforcement for the undesirable behavior.
Respond (confront) with reality when M.J.B. makes unrealistic statements such as "I've stopped vomiting so there's nothing really wrong with me."	Provides constructive feedback about how improving nutrition will give her energy to look at other aspects of her life so that food will not be so all-consuming. Patient needs to be confronted because she denies the psychologic aspects of her situation and often expresses a sense of inadequacy and depression.
Be aware of own	Feelings of disgust,

reaction to M.J.B.'s behavior. Avoid arguing.	hostility, and infuriation are not uncommon when caring for these patients. Prognosis remains poor even with stabilization of weight as other problems may remain. Many patients continue to see themselves as fat, and there is also a high incidence of affective disorders, social phobias, obsessive–compulsive symptoms, substance abuse, and psychosexual dysfunction. The staff needs to deal with own responses/feelings so they do not interfere with care of the patient.
Encourage M.J.B. to recognize positive characteristics related to self.	Discussion of positive aspects of the self system, such as social skills, work abilities, education, talents, and appearance can reinforce patient's feelings of being a worthwhile/competent person.

Actions/Interventions	Rationale
Assist M.J.B. to assume control in areas other than dieting/weight loss (e.g., management of own daily activities, work/leisure choices).	Feelings of personal ineffectiveness, low self-esteem, and perfectionism are often part of the problem. Patient feels helpless to change, and requires assistance to problem-solve methods of control in life situations.
Help M.J.B. formulate goals for self not related to eating (e.g., choice of a satisfying vocation/avocation and formulation of a manageable plan to reach those goals, one at a time on a short-/long-term basis as appropriate).	Patient needs to recognize ability to control other areas in life and may need to learn problem-solving skills in order to achieve this control. Patient may not know how to set realistic goals and choices may be influenced by altered thought processes.
Assist M.J.B. to confront sexual fears. Provide sex education as necessary.	Major physical/psychologic changes in adolescence can contribute to development of this problem. Feelings of powerlessness and loss of control of feelings (in

	particular sexual), sensations, and physical development lead to an unconscious desire to de-sexualize self. Patient often believes that these fears can be overcome by taking control of bodily appearance/ development/ function.
Encourage M.J.B. to take charge of her own life in a more healthful way by making her own decisions and accepting herself as she is.	Patient often doesn't know what she may want for self. Parents (mother) made decisions for her.
Encourage acceptance of inadequacies as well as strengths. Let M.J.B. know that it is acceptable to be different from family, particularly mother.	Patient also believes she has to be the best in everything and holds self responsible for being perfect. She needs to develop a sense of control in other ways, besides dieting and weight loss.
Involve in personal development program.	Learning about proper application of makeup and other methods of

Actions/Interventions	Rationale
	enhancing personal appearance may be helpful to long-range sense of self-esteem.
Use interpersonal psychotherapy rather than interpretive therapy.	More helpful for the patient to discover feelings/impulses/needs from within own self. Patient has not learned this internal control as a child.
Encourage M.J.B. to express anger and acknowledge when it is verbalized.	Important to know that anger is part of self and as such is acceptable. Expressing anger may need to be taught to patient, as anger is generally considered unacceptable in the family and therefore patient does not express it.
Assist M.J.B. to learn strategies other than eating for dealing with feelings. Have M.J.B. keep a diary of feelings, particularly when thinking about food.	Feelings are the underlying issue, and patients often use food instead of dealing with feelings appropriately. May need to learn to recognize feelings

	and how to express them in a positive manner.
Assess feelings of helplessness/ hopelessness.	Fifty-four percent of patients with anorexia have a history of major affective disorder; thirty-three percent have a history of minor affective disorder.
Be alert to suicidal ideation/behavior.	Intensity of anxiety/ panic about weight gain, depression, hopeless feelings may lead to suicidal attempts, particularly if patient is impulsive.
Involve in group therapy.	Provides an opportunity to talk about feelings and try out new behaviors.

PATIENT PROBLEM STATEMENT/ FOCUS (NURSING DIAGNOSIS)

Knowledge deficit [learning need] related to learned maladaptive coping skills and lack of exposure to/unfamiliarity with information about condition evidenced by verbalization of misconception of relationship of behaviors (preoccupation with extreme fear of obesity and distortion of own body image; refusal to eat, bingeing and purging; and current hospitalization), and request for new information and expressions of desire to learn more adaptive ways of coping with stressors.

PATIENT OUTCOMES/ EVALUATION CRITERIA

Short-term:
• Identifies relationship of signs/symptoms (weight loss, tooth decay, skin problems) to behaviors of not eating/binge–purging within 3 days (3 PM 6/26).
• Assumes responsibility for own learning within 2 weeks (7/6).
Intermediate:
• Verbalizes awareness of and plans for lifestyle changes to maintain normal weight without aberrant eating pattern within 2 weeks (7/6).
Long-term:
• Displays no preventable complications at 3 to 6 month check.

Actions/Interventions	Rationale
Determine level of knowledge and readiness to learn.	Learning is easier when it begins where the learner is.
Note blocks to learning (e.g., physical/ intellectual/ emotional).	Malnutrition, family problems, affective disorders, obsessive-compulsive symptoms can be blocks to learning.
Review dietary needs, answering questions as indicated.	May need assistance with planning for new way of eating.

Provide information about and encourage the use of relaxation and other stress management techniques.

New ways of coping with feelings of anxiety and fear will help patient to manage these feelings in more effective ways, assisting in giving up maladaptive behaviors of not eating/bingeing–purging.

Assist with establishing a sensible exercise program. Caution regarding overexercise.

Exercise can assist with developing a positive body image and combats depression. Excessive exercise increases caloric needs/weight loss.

Review appropriate skin-care needs. Encourage bathing every other day. Use skin cream twice a day and after bathing; massage skin, especially over bony prominences. Observe for reddened/blanched areas.

Frequent baths contribute to dryness of the skin. Supplemental lubrication of the skin decreases itching/flaking and reduces potential for breakdown. Massage enhances circulation to the skin and improves skin tone. Involves patient in monitoring and intervening in own therapy.

Actions/Interventions	Rationale
Stress importance of adequate nutrition/ fluid intake.	Improved nutrition can improve thinking processes, skin condition, activity tolerance, and sense of general well-being.
Provide written information for M.J.B.	Helpful as reminder of and reinforcement for learning.
Encourage M.J.B. to ask caring friends and coworkers to provide support for necessary changes.	Can serve as a support system to help patient make necessary lifestyle changes.
Refer for dental consult/care. Establish plan for routine dental follow-up care.	Purging behavior (stomach acids) damages gum tissues and tooth enamel. Poor dentition affects proper intake of desired foods.
Refer to National Association of Anorexia Nervosa and Associated Disorders.	May be a helpful source of support and information for patient and significant other(s).

PEDIATRIC/ADOLESCENT PATIENT SITUATION: ASTHMA

N.W. presented at Clinic at 1445 in acute asthma attack. She received epinephrine 0.3 mg SQ at 1455 and repeated at 1520. Patient reported moderate improvement in dyspnea.

Transferred by wheelchair to medical floor and admitted.

ADMITTING PHYSICIAN'S ORDERS

ABGs, CBC, electrolytes, serum theophylline level, CXR stat.
Repeat ABGs in 6 hr.
IV D5 ½ NS at 100 cc/hr × 4 hr then 50 cc/hr.
Aminophylline 250 mg IV stat (start after lab drawn), then 40 mg/hr continuous.
IPPB stat and q 2 hr with Bronkosol 0.5 ml in 3 ml saline.
O_2 4L/prongs.
Solu-Cortef 250 mg IV stat, 100 mg IV q 6 hr × 5.
Diet/activity as tolerated.
Instruct in decreasing dosage of prednisone and use of cromolyn in preparation for discharge.

NURSING HISTORY and ASSESSMENT

Name: N.W. Informant: Patient and mother
Reliability (scale 1–4): 4
Age: 17 DOB: 2/4/68
Sex: Female Race: Native American
Admission date: 11/12/85 From: Clinic/per wheelchair Time: 1540

ACTIVITY/REST

Subjective

Occupation: Student/sales clerk, 2 evenings/week and weekends

Usual activities/hobbies: Watch some TV, listen to music
Leisure-time activities: "Don't have any now"
Limitations imposed by illness: Generally sedentary; has occasional dyspnea after exercise/strenuous activity
Sleep: Hours: Some nights 10–12, others 3–4
Naps: -0- Aids: None
Insomnia: Reports occasionally wakens early (2–4 AM) and unable to get back to sleep. Related to: Dyspnea/studying/sometimes "too tired to sleep, worry about school/boyfriend"
Rested upon awakening: Not always

Objective

Observed response to activity: Cardiovascular: Tachycardia (postadrenalin) Respiratory: Increased dyspnea with activity/speech currently.
Mental status: Restless, anxious
Muscle mass/tone: Underdeveloped/thin; normal
Posture: Leaning forward
Tremors: Hands (postadrenalin)
ROM: Full Strength: Good Deformity: -0-

CIRCULATION

Subjective

History of elevated BP: -0- Heart trouble: -0-
Ankle edema: -0-
Extremities: Numbness/tingling: -0-
Claudication: -0- Slow healing: -0-
Cough/character of sputum: Tight, nonproductive
Change in frequency/amount of urine: No

Objective

BP: R: Sit: 122/66 Lying: Too dyspneac
Stand: Deferred
L: Sit: 118/64 Lying: Too dyspneac
Stand: Deferred
Pulse pressure: 54–56
Pulse: Apical: 110 Radial: 110 Quality: 4+ (Postadrenalin)
Heart sounds: normal S_1, S_2; palpable through chest wall/normal PMI
Rub/murmur: No Rhythm: Regular
Chest sounds: Bilateral wheezing and diminished bases
Jugular vein distention: Full bilateral with strong pulse
Peripheral pulses: Equal all extremities +4
Capillary refill: Brisk, less than 3 seconds
Temperature of extremities: Warm/equal
Homan's sign: Negative
Distribution and quality of hair: Shaves legs
Color: Skin: pale, face flushed
Mucous membranes/lips: Slightly cyanotic
Nailbeds: Dusky, biting evident with cuticles red/inflamed
Conjunctiva: Clear Sclera: White

EGO INTEGRITY

Subjective

Report of stress factors: "My life's falling apart. I'm failing algebra, I broke up with my boyfriend. I have trouble studying and working both, but since Dad died, we need the money."
Ways of handling stress: "I try to forget my problems and just keep going."
Financial concerns: Limited resources. (Widowed mother works in dry cleaning store, receives Social Security for dependent children.)

Relationship status: Recently broke up with boyfriend
Cultural factors: Late adolescent, lower socioeconomic, Native American
Religion: Methodist, not practicing currently, "works on Sundays"
Lifestyle: "Not enough money, food, or time for anything"
Recent changes: Declined with father's death 2 years ago

Objective

Emotional status: Anxious, restive, irritable, possible depression
Observed physiologic response(s): Tearful, "rocking," twisting tissue in hands

ELIMINATION

Subjective

Usual bowel pattern: Every 1 or 2 days
Last BM: This AM Character of stool: Hard formed/brown color today
Bleeding/diarrhea/constipation: -0- Laxative used: None
Usual voiding pattern: q 4–5 times per day.
Pain/burning/difficulty with urination: None
Character of urine: Clear, amber

Objective

Abdomen tender: Upper L/R quadrant
Soft/firm: Soft
Palpable mass: -0- Bowel sounds: Active all 4 quadrants

Size/girth: Not done
Palpate bladder: Deferred, unable to recline

FOOD/FLUID

Subjective

Special diet (type): "Regular for age"
Dietary pattern: Breakfast: Rarely
Lunch: Sandwich/fast food
Dinner: Balanced meal four times per week when eats at home. Usual beverage: Coffee 1–2 cups/day, diet colas, iced tea
Last meal/intake: Last PM—meat, potato, salad. Fluids only today.
Loss of appetite: During attacks Nausea: With asthma medications
Vomiting: -0-
Heartburn/indigestion: -0- Allergy/food intolerance: -0-
Mastication/swallowing problems: no
Usual wt: 140 lb Changes in weight: About 10 lb decrease in last 6 months
Diuretic therapy: -0-

Objective

Current weight: 132 lb/60.0 kg Ht: 5′10″
Body build: Thin/willowy
Skin turgor: Good Mucous membranes: Dry
Edema: -0- Jugular distention: -0-
Condition of teeth/gums: Intact, denies dental problems
Halitosis: -0-
Appearance of tongue: Dry/red
Mucous membranes: Intact
Bowel sounds: Active all 4 quadrants
Breath sounds: Bilateral wheeze/diminished bases

HYGIENE

Subjective

Activities of daily living: Independent in all areas

Objective

General appearance: Clean/dressed appropriately for weather, no makeup or jewelry, hair cut short/straight, nails down to quick, skin dry/flaky.

NEUROSENSORY

Subjective

Fainting spells/dizziness: -0- Headaches: 2–3 times per week
Stroke: -0- Weakness/tingling/numbness: -0-
Seizures: -0-
Eyes/vision loss: Nearsighted/no recent change noted
Last eye exam 1 year ago Glaucoma: -0-
Cataract: -0-

Objective

Mental status: Alert, oriented to time, place, person
Delusions: -0- Hallucinations: -0-
Affect: Anxious/tense
Memory recent/remote: Intact
Pupil reaction: PERLA Contacts: In place
Handgrips/release: Equal/medium, tremulous
Speech: Clear but weak/breathy

Unusual speech pattern/impairment: Short responses of 3–4 words related to dyspnea.

PAIN/COMFORT

Subjective

Location: Headache, temples, bilateral Intensity (scale 1–10): 5–6
Quality; Dull ache Frequency: 2–3 times per week Duration: Several hours
Precipitating factors: "Sometimes wake up with it," "when things get too hectic"
How relieved: 3 tablets ASA, lies down with cool cloth over eyes

Objective

No headache at present to observe
Narrowed focus: Currently focused on work of breathing

RESPIRATION

Subjective

Dyspnea (related to): "Asthma, chest gets tight and I can't cough up the mucus."
Cough: Tight/nonproductive
Emphysema: -0- Bronchitis: -0- Asthma: × 6 years
Smoker: -0- packs/day: -0-/occasional marijuana "once or twice a week"
Use of respiratory aids: Prescription inhaler

Objective

Respiratory rate: 34
Depth and quality: Shallow inspiration/prolonged expiration phase

Breath sounds: Diffuse bilateral wheezes with diminished bases

Use of accessory muscles: Leaning forward with mild intercostal retraction   Nasal flaring: Moderate with inspiration. Pursed-lip exhalation noted.

Cyanosis: Lips/nails dusky   Clubbing of fingers: -0-

Sputum characteristics: Cough nonproductive

Mentation/restlessness: Alert/anxious/restless, rocking upper torso and squeezing hands

SAFETY

Subjective

Blood transfusions: None

History of sexually transmitted disease: -0-

Allergies: Penicillin; pollens/animal dander
  Reactions: Rash; wheezing, respiratory distress

History of accidental injuries: -0-

Vision impaired: Corrected
  Hearing impaired: -0-

Expressions of ideation of violence (self/others): -0-

Objective

Temperature: 99°F PO

Skin integrity: Good   Rashes: -0-

Sores: -0-   Bruises: -0-

Scars: RLQ, appendectomy

Strength (general): Normal/equal bilateral

Muscle tone: Normal, hand tremors after adrenalin

ROM: Full, all extremities and neck

Gait: Halting/unsteady at present
  Paresthesia: -0-   Paralysis: -0-

SEXUALITY Female:

Subjective

Last menstrual period: just finished
Duration: 4 days
Frequency: Average 28 days
Vaginal discharge: -0- Age at menarche: 12 yr
Practice breast self-exam: Not routinely
Last PAP smear: 9 months ago Complaints: -0-
Method of birth control: Pill
Pregnancy concerns: None
Sexually active: Yes Condom use: No

Objective

Vaginal exam: Not done Breast: Well developed, exam deferred

SOCIAL INTERACTIONS

Subjective

Marital status: Single Living with: Mother; brother, age 15 yr; sister age 12 yr
Extended family: Infrequent contact with uncle living out of state
Other: Some friends school/neighborhood, but "doesn't have time to socialize"
Role within family structure: Oldest sibling/child
Report of problems: "We really don't see each other, except at dinner because we're all so busy"
Coping behaviors: "I handle it myself and try not to bother others"
Frequency of social contacts: "Don't go out like I used to"

Objective

Verbal/nonverbal communication with family/significant other(s): Holding mother's hand
Family interaction patterns: Mother patting N.W.'s arm, repeating "everything will be OK"

TEACHING/LEARNING

Subjective

Dominant language: English
Level of education: High school senior
Learning disabilities: -0-
Familial risk factors (indicate relationship):
Cancer: -0- Stroke: -0-
Diabetes: Maternal great-aunt and grandmother
Heart disease: Father died MI, 1983, age 40 yr/ paternal grandparents died before age 65 yr, CV disease High BP: Father
Kidney disease: -0- Other: Tuberculosis—uncle, 1982
Health beliefs/practices: "Nothing particular, doesn't think about it much"
Special health-care practices: None
Routine medications as stated by patient:

Drug:	*Dose:*	*Schedule:*	*Time/last dose:*
Bronkometer	2 inhalations	q 4 hr prn	2:15 PM
Theo-Dur	200 mg	qid	12 noon
Terbutaline	2.5 mg	tid	Stopped taking about a week ago due to "nausea/shakes"
Birth control	1	daily	this AM

Does patient take medications regularly?: All except terbutaline

Nonprescription (OTC/street) drugs: Occasional ASA/occasional marijuana

Use of alcohol (amount/frequency): Social, occasional beer

Admitting diagnosis (physician): Acute asthma attack, recurrent with need for IV aminophylline/Solu-Cortef

Reason for hospitalization (patient): "Can't get my breath"

History of current complaint: "Attack began about 7:30 AM while getting ready for school; my inhaler didn't help, I just got worse, so I went to the clinic"

Patient expectations of this hospitalization: "Breathe better and stop these asthma attacks. Doctor says he's going to change my medicine."

Other relevant illness and/or previous hospitalizations/surgeries: 1–2 admissions per year for asthma; 3 in the past year. Appendectomy at age 10 yr

Evidence of failure to improve: Fourth hospitalization this year; last one, 3 weeks ago

Last physical exam: Complete exam 9 months ago/respiratory workup 3 weeks ago

DISCHARGE PLAN CONSIDERATIONS

Data obtained: 11/12/85 Anticipated discharge: 11/15/85

Resources available: Persons: Mother
Financial: Limited

Anticipated change in home situation or need for assistance: Will need help with finances

PEDIATRIC/ADOLESCENT NURSING CARE PLAN: ASTHMA

PATIENT PROBLEM STATEMENT/ FOCUS (NURSING DIAGNOSIS)

Airway clearance, ineffective related to bronchial muscle spasm and retained secretions evidenced by dyspnea, bilateral expiratory wheeze, prolonged expiratory phase, tachypnea, and cyanosis.

PATIENT OUTCOMES/ EVALUATION CRITERIA

- Demonstrates decreased respiratory rate and work of breathing within 12 hours (0400 11/13).
- Readily expectorates secretions and expiratory wheeze clears within 48 hours (1600 11/14).

Actions/Interventions	Rationale
Place in high Fowler's or orthopneic position.	Position of most effective lung expansion.
Encourage use of pursed-lip breathing.	Creates positive-end expiratory pressure to minimize collapse of airways.
Administer O_2 at 4 L per nasal prongs.	Bronchodilator enhances pulmonary blood flow before relaxing bronchial spasm, creating transient fall in PO_2 (ventilation/ perfusion

	mismatch), which can be minimized by supplemental O_2.
Assess respiratory status q hr and prn; include rate, work of breathing, use of accessory muscles, cyanosis, cough, sputum production, and breath sounds.	Initial parameters serve as baseline for noting improvement/ deterioration and evaluation of therapy.
Administer IV fluids D5 ½ NS, 100 cc/hr × 4, at 8 PM decrease to 50 cc/hr. Encourage PO fluids; 1500 cc minimum.	Corrects dehydration and liquefies secretions enhancing expectoration.
Provide more warm fluids than cold.	Decreases spasms and facilitates expectoration.
Monitor intake/output.	Overcorrection of dehydration may result in intrapulmonary fluid shifts.
Administer aminophyllin loading dose: 250 mg IV over 20 minutes, then: Maintenance therapy: continuous infusion of 40 mg/hr.	Bronchodilator decreases bronchospasm by relaxing bronchial smooth muscle.
Monitor BP and pulse	Potential side effects

Actions/Interventions	Rationale
q 5 minutes during loading dose then q hr and prn.	include hypotension, palpitations, and cardiac dysrhythmias.
Administer Bronkosol 0.5 ml in 3 cc NS via IPPB q 2 hr.	Provides delivery of inhaled bronchodilator when patient is unable to take in adequate inspiration or use metered-dose inhaler/hand-held nebulizer.
Monitor pulse before, during, and after treatment.	Side effect of tachycardia may require alteration/ discontinuation of therapy.
Administer Solu-Cortef loading dose: 250 mg IV stat. Maintenance dose: 100 mg IV q 6 hr × 5, starting at 10 PM.	Decreases bronchial inflammation, reducing airway obstruction.
Monitor/graph serial ABG results.	Provides readily accessible record of respiratory status/ effectiveness of therapy.

PATIENT PROBLEM STATEMENT/ FOCUS (NURSING DIAGNOSIS)

Anxiety moderate related to perceived threat of death (difficulty breathing) evidenced by apprehension, restlessness, increased tension (posture), and focus on self.

PATIENT OUTCOMES/ EVALUATION CRITERIA

- Reports anxiety related to physiologic factors reduced to a manageable level within 12 hours (1500 11/13).

Actions/Interventions	Rationale
Assess respiratory status in presence of increasing anxiety.	Anxiety may reflect physiologic deterioration.
Encourage pursed-lip breathing.	Assists patient to "take control" of respiratory situation.
Provide quiet environment and maintain calm, confident manner.	Promotes rest/relaxation.
Coordinate interventions/ activities to allow for periods of undisturbed rest.	Activity increases O_2 requirements and may heighten anxiety.
Acknowledge fearful situation.	Physiologic anxiety is fearful and it is

	helpful to let the patient know it is all right to express the fear. Other anxieties are overshadowed by breathing problem.

PATIENT PROBLEM STATEMENT/ FOCUS (NURSING DIAGNOSIS)

Coping ineffective, individual related to family/ social/situational crisis, personal vulnerability, work overload, inadequate coping skills as evidenced by frequent headaches, inability to sleep, difficulty studying and recurrent exacerbations of asthma.

PATIENT OUTCOMES/EVALUATION

- Verbalizes awareness of source(s) of anxiety within 24 hours (1600 11/3).
- Demonstrates initial problem-solving skills within 72 hours (1600 11/15).

Actions/Interventions	Rationale
Assess level of anxiety and N.W.'s perception of her situation.	Important to developing plan of care and need for further assistance.
Note verbal/nonverbal behaviors indicating anxiety.	Confirm/substantiate presence of problems that may require intervention.

Identify coping mechanisms N.W. is currently using. Encourage verbalization, allow expressions of feelings of denial, depression, and anger. Assure N.W. that these are normal feelings.

Frequency of hospital admissions during past 12 months and patient's expressions of despair and hopelessness are indicators of possible ineffective coping/unresolved grieving, which may require more in-depth counseling/intervention.

Be available for listening and talking while performing necessary tasks.

Establishes rapport and allows patient to express feelings/concerns in an accepting atmosphere.

Discuss and refer to appropriate resources for help (e.g., social worker, counseling).

Although patient may already have information about some resources, may need additional information/support to resolve problems that are contributing to readmission to the hospital.

PATIENT PROBLEM STATEMENT/ FOCUS (NURSING DIAGNOSIS)

Knowledge deficit related to lack of understanding about interrelationship of disease process, contributing factors, and therapies and evidenced by recurrent asthmatic episodes, discontinuing medication without seeking advice, and exposure to potential risk factors.

PATIENT OUTCOMES/ EVALUATION CRITERIA

- Assesses activities/environment and identifies factors contributing to exacerbation of symptoms within 48 hours (1600 11/14).
- Demonstrates proper administration of Prednisone and cromolyn within 72 hours (1600 11/15)/ or before discharge.

Actions/Interventions	Rationale
Assess current level of knowledge.	Patient has been living with this disease for 6 years. Information about how she perceives the situation will help the nurse provide/reinforce information and correct misconceptions.
Discuss effects of caffeine and marijuana on the body and respiratory system.	Both drugs are stimulants that increase catecholamine release in the body, indicating a stress situation. In addition, numerous chemicals in marijuana may act as allergens,

	precipitating an allergic reaction/asthma.
Identify noncaffeinated beverage choices to meet daily fluid needs.	May require up to 3000 cc/day to maintain hydration, liquefy secretions, and offset diuretic effect of theophylline.
Recommend use of acetaminophen instead of ASA for pain relief.	ASA may precipitate asthma attack.
Review relaxation techniques/stress management program matched to her individual needs.	Stress reduction can help reduce/minimize headaches as well as asthma attacks.
Instruct N.W./mother in protocol of oral Prednisone and cromolyn sodium spinhaler use.	Information necessary to promote accurate self-care behaviors.
Explain use and side effects as well as results of omitting medication.	Knowledge/understanding may enhance cooperation with therapeutic regimen and reduce frequency of attacks.
Provide written instructions outlining correct	Provides post-discharge reinforcement of

Actions/Interventions	Rationale
use of spinhaler.	inpatient instruction.
Have N.W. repeat instructions.	Patient's repetition reveals depth of understanding, but not necessarily commitment to follow-through.
Discuss the need/ importance for N.W. to assume responsibility for her own wellness by recognition of early signs/symptoms of developing attack and timely seeking of medical advice.	Encourages patient to form a commitment to wellness.
Review dietary and stress reduction needs to support the immune system.	Poor nutrition as well as stress in general may weaken the immune system, which may contribute to exacerbation of asthma attacks.
Identify potential health risks (e.g., familial history of diabetes, hypertension, heart disease; and unprotected sexual	Promotes awareness and participation in responsibility of own preventive health care.

activity). Refer to appropriate informational resources.

ALTERNATE HEALTH-CARE SETTING PATIENT SITUATION: INDEPENDENT PSYCHIATRIC NURSING PRACTICE

Mrs. M.B. has been in therapy for the past 4 years with a psychologist and has now been referred to the psychiatric nurse clinical specialist for help with understanding male sexuality.

Name: Mrs. M.B. Age: 42 DOB: 3/15/45
Sex: Female Race: Caucasion
Admission date: 6/3/87 Time: 1100
Source of information: client Reliability (Scale 1–4): 4
Family member/significant other(s): daughter, age 13 yr

NURSING HISTORY and ASSESSMENT

ACTIVITY/REST

Subjective

Occupation: Beautician
Usual activities/hobbies: Works long hours; skis, "when I can get away"
Leisure-time activities: Reads, attends personal growth workshops
Limitations imposed by condition: None
Sleep: Hours: 5–6 Naps: None
Sleep aids: Occasional glass of wine to relax
Insomnia: occasionally wakens early (0300–0400) and "spin my wheels worrying about things"
Rested upon awakening: Not usually

Objective

 Mental status: Alert, slightly hypervigilant

CIRCULATION

Subjective

No history of hypertension, heart trouble, swelling of ankles, phlebitis, or slow healing
No cough

Objective

BP: 136/88 Pulse (radial): 92

EGO INTEGRITY

Subjective

What kind of a person are you?: "Hyperactive, usually positive but lose my temper quickly"
What do you think of your body?: "Not much. Wish I were thinner. I've been working on improving my skin and want to have some plastic surgery on my eyes and neck when I can afford it."
How would you rate your self-esteem: 3 on a 1–10 scale
What are your moods?: Depressed, guilty, anxious
Are you a nervous person?: Yes
Are your feelings easily hurt?: Somewhat
Stress factors: Relationship with significant other; trying to build business and "keep head above water"
Previous patterns of coping with stress: Loses temper easily and throws things; also blames self and feels guilty
Financial concerns: Worries about business making money but otherwise OK with money from late husband's estate
Relationship status: Four-year involvement with

current partner. States they "fight a lot." Previously married: Yes, for 14 yr
Cultural factors: Grew up in small, southeastern town
Lifestyle: Middle-class, establishing own business
Significant losses/changes: Husband's death 6 years ago
Stage of grief/manifestations of loss: Continues to feel sadness, anger, and guilt about husband's death
Religion: Was raised in the Baptist church but doesn't attend presently

Objective

Emotional status: presents with a calm, friendly, manner. Cooperative. Moving hands and jiggling legs frequently. Moves restlessly in chair from time to time.
Verbal/nonverbal behavior is congruent. Speech is well-modulated.
Defense mechanisms: Uses denial, rationalization and projection, and is passive-aggressive

ELIMINATION

Subjective

States no unusual problems noted

Objective

Deferred

FOOD/FLUID

Subjective

Usual diet: Doesn't eat breakfast and usually eats lunch on the run. Tries to have regular meal at night with her daughter.
Usual weight: 140 lb

Objective

Current weight: 138 lb   Height: 5′6″
Body build: mesomorph

HYGIENE

Subjective

Independent in activities of daily living

Objective

Well-dressed, stylish clothing; hair arranged in a becoming style, clean and neat.

NEUROSENSORY

Subjective

Headaches: Occasional migraines (1–2/month)
Eyes: Wears glasses to read fine print

Objective

Mental status:
Oriented to time, place, and person
Cooperative

Memory intact for immediate, recent, and remote events
Intellectual functioning: Fund of information and vocabulary appear appropriate for educational level (post–high school)
Judgment: Demonstrates unimpaired ability to compare and evaluate facts, ideas, and choices and draw appropriate conclusions
Comprehension: Average performance on serial sevens test
Thought processes: patterns of speech: Normal rate and flow. No evidence of hallucinations or delusions.

Speech: Clear, intelligible
Mood: Sad, anxious
Affect: Appropriate, anxious
Displays insight about current problems
Wears glasses to read

PAIN/COMFORT

Subjective

Only when migraine headaches occur, once or twice per month, lasting 1–2 days
Precipitating factors: Related to stress
Takes a "shot of Demerol" to relieve migraine when other measures fail (e.g., bedrest, relaxation tapes, and biofeedback), "goes home and sleeps it off."

Objective

Emotional response: Appropriate to situation

SAFETY

Subjective

Vision: Wears glasses for astigmatism
Expresses some fear of hurting others when she becomes "so angry"

Objective

No abnormalities noted

SEXUALITY FEMALE:

Subjective

Sexual orientation: Heterosexual
Sexual concerns: Expresses concern that mate may molest her daughter. Has become aware through therapy that she was molested by a family friend when she was 11 yr of age
Age at menarche: 12 yr Hysterectomy 4 years ago (excessive bleeding). No hormones taken.

Objective

Deferred

SOCIAL INTERACTIONS

Subjective

Memory of early years: Has recently become aware of incident where male family friend molested her at age 11 yr. Unhappy relationship with sisters, one older, one younger, while growing up.

Relationship status: Living with man last 4 yr
Genogram: To be done 6/10/87
Family dynamics: Love/hate relationship with partner. Says he puts her down, tells her she is not a capable person, then she gets angry, throws things. Teen-aged daughter does not have a positive relationship with mother's mate. Mother and daughter have a fairly good relationship with occasional clashes over mate.
Extended family: Older sister lives in area; younger sister and mother live out of state
Other support persons: G., younger woman who works with her
Role within family structure: Mother, wage-earner, mate
Report of problems: See presenting information
Coping behaviors: Withdraws, migraine headaches, precipitates a crisis, then becomes angry and occasionally throws things
Frequency of social contacts: 2–3 times a week, movie with friends, activities with daughter, she and mate go out occasionally

Objective

Verbal/nonverbal communications with family/significant other(s): Not observed
Family interaction pattern: Not observed

TEACHING/LEARNING

Subjective

Dominant language: English
Education level: 3 yr post–high school. Some college.
Cognitive limitations: Some difficulty with memory

and retention of class work in school. Believes does not process information well.

Health beliefs/practices: States she is interested in self-growth activities, attends workshops

Special health-care practices: Takes vitamins daily

Familial risk factors:

Father died of lung cancer 10 years ago.

Maternal grandmother had high blood pressure.

Mother has been an alcoholic.

Prescribed medications:

Desyrel 50 mg 0600, 1400, and 2000 Takes regularly for anxiety

Nonprescription drugs: OTC: occasionally takes aspirin/acetaminophen for headache; states she does not use street drugs; reports use of alcohol on social occasions, 1–2 highballs

Admitting diagnosis (physician): DSM III-R:

Axis I 300.02 Generalized Anxiety

Axis II: Dependent Personality

Axis III: Cluster Headaches

Axis IV: Stressors: new business, relationship problems with men

Axis V: Moderate

Reason for entry into health-care system: Extreme anxiety, prolonged grief over husband's death, and conflict in current relationship

Client expectations of treatment: "Would like to learn to manage anger more effectively, come to a resolution of current relationship, and to deal with recent awareness of childhood incident of sexual abuse"

Evidence of failure to improve: Has been in therapy for the past 4 years, believes she has learned some things but needs to become more self-sufficient

Last complete physical exam: 6 months ago by family physician, Dr. Jones.

DISCHARGE PLAN CONSIDERATIONS

Anticipated date of discharge from care: 6 months
Resources available: Had difficulty identifying people she can rely on for help when she is distressed
Normal financial concerns, has insurance, which will pay for therapy
No changes anticipated in living situation

ALTERNATE HEALTH-CARE SETTING CARE PLAN: INDEPENDENT PSYCHIATRIC NURSING

CLIENT PROBLEM STATEMENT/ FOCUS (NURSING DIAGNOSIS)

Anxiety, moderate related to threat to self-concept and interaction patterns evidenced by expressions of concern about the relationship between her daughter and her mate, extraneous movements of her body, and poor eye contact.

CLIENT OUTCOMES/EVALUATION CRITERIA

Short-term:
- Verbalizes reduction of anxiety (by the sixth session).

Long-term:
- Sits calmly without extraneous movements (within 6 months).

Actions/Interventions	Rationale
Establish and maintain a trusting relationship through use of warmth, empathy, and respect. Provide adequate time for response. Communicate support of self-expression.	Attending behaviors can increase the degree of comfort the client experiences with the nurse, decreasing anxious feelings and promoting therapeutic communication.
Determine how M.B. is currently	Provides information about what is being

Actions/Interventions	Rationale
managing anxiety.	helpful and identifies needs for further intervention.
Have M.B. identify and describe the sensations of emotional and physical feelings. Help M.B. to link behavior and feelings. Validate inferences and assumptions with M.B.	In order to adopt new coping responses, the client first needs to recognize anxiety and be aware of feelings, how they link to certain maladaptive coping responses, and own responsibility in learning to control behavior.
Help M.B. to recognize precursors of angry outbursts and discuss ways to deal with feelings in more positive ways. Encourage M.B. to maintain a journal, focusing on feelings and events as they occur.	Early recognition enables client to diminish anxious feelings, maintain control, and prevent outbursts. Writing serves to decrease the anxiety while learning about it.
Identify and explore conflictual issues by beginning with nonthreatening topics and progressing to more conflict-laden ones.	Beginning with simple topics promotes comfort level, decreases anxiety, and increases sense of success and progress.

Explore how M.B. has dealt with anxiety in the past and what methods produced relief. Help to identify the maladaptive effects of present coping responses.	Analyzing coping mechanisms used previously, identifying available resources, and accepting personal responsibility for change promotes learning new, adaptive coping responses.
Demonstrate and encourage use of relaxation techniques, meditation, biofeedback, and visualization.	Stress management brings about a decreased heart rate, lowers metabolism, and decreases respiration. The relaxation response is the physiologic opposite of the anxiety response.
Develop a regular physical activity program, aerobics three times a week, use of 10-minute energy walk when she feels stressed.	Excess energy is discharged in a healthful manner and biochemical effects of exercise decrease feelings of anxiety.
Review use of Desyrel 50 mg.	Anti-anxiety medication provides relief from the immobilizing effects of anxiety while freeing client to work on new coping skills.

CLIENT PROBLEM STATEMENT/ FOCUS (NURSING DIAGNOSIS)

Self-esteem disturbance related to lack of belief in her own ability to make decisions and be successful, evidenced by lack of eye contact and repeated questioning—"Is that right?"

CLIENT OUTCOMES/EVALUATION CRITERIA

Short-term:
- Acknowledges feelings of low self-esteem (first session).

Intermediate:
- Demonstrates increased self-esteem by expressions of sense of well-being, satisfaction with self (within 3 months).

Long-term:
- Makes decisions without asking another person for their opinion (within 6 months).

Actions/Interventions	Rationale
Meet once a week for 50-minute session using insight-oriented psychotherapy, transactional analysis, and gestalt. Instruct M.B. to read *Born to Win*.	Becoming aware of reasons for behaviors and beliefs provides the first step for change and these tools provide information/ opportunity to initiate change.
Convey unconditional positive regard by Active-listening,	Unconditional acceptance of an individual serves to

assisting with development of problem-solving skills, and attending behaviors.	counteract feelings of worthlessness by reinforcing that she is worthy of another person's respect.
Encourage and support M.B. in learning to trust own feelings and make own decisions.	Recognition and positive reinforcement enhance self-esteem and encourage repetition of desirable behaviors.
Encourage independence in own responsibilities and decision making and acceptance of possibility of failure.	Promotes sense of encouragement and positive self-esteem. Taking risk of failure enhances confidence in ability to manage/control consequences of own actions.
Discuss problem of alcoholism in family and how it affected relationships among the family members.	Recognition of the ways in which mother's drinking impacted on the development of her self-esteem/relationships with others as an adult provides opportunity for her to make positive changes.
Encourage attendance in Children of Alcoholics group.	Participation in these group activities can provide support and a sense of not being

Actions/Interventions	Rationale
	alone as well as providing information about the problems related to growing up in an alcoholic family.
Assist M.B. in setting realistic goals of her own.	Tends to do what others want, ignores own wishes, needs to learn to trust herself.

CLIENT PROBLEM STATEMENT/ FOCUS (NURSING DIAGNOSIS)

Grieving, dysfunctional related to lack of resolution of the grief and guilt over her perceived role in her husband's death as evidenced by statements such as "I should have been there and it wouldn't have happened."

CLIENT OUTCOMES/EVALUATION CRITERIA

Short-term:
- Discusses feelings of responsibility and guilt regarding husband's death (by second session).

Intermediate:
- Reports awareness that she does not need to feel guilty about being away when her husband died (within 2 months).

Long-term:
- Completes the grieving process for him by

acknowledging his role and responsibility in his own death (within 6 months).

Actions/Interventions	Rationale
Note verbal/nonverbal expressions of guilt and self-blame.	Identification of grief thoughts and behaviors provides information for appropriate interventions.
Identify avoidance behaviors, (e.g., anger, withdrawal).	Recognition can help with beginning a new approach to resolving feelings that have been ignored.
Discuss reality of not being present when husband died and that he chose to continue to live his life independently.	Acceptance of own powerlessness to have prevented husband's death and his part in the event provides opportunity for resolution.
Encourage verbalization and acceptance of feelings as "normal."	Promotes acceptance of own feelings.
Identify and reinforce use of previously effective coping skills.	Identification of helpful ways client is already dealing with problems allows client to feel positive about self.

CLIENT PROBLEM STATEMENT/ FOCUS (NURSING DIAGNOSIS)

Sexual dysfunction related to ineffective role modeling by her parents, lack of knowledge about male sexuality, and incident of sexual abuse in own childhood evidenced by expressions of concern, questions, and willingness to discuss sexual issues.

CLIENT OUTCOMES/EVALUATION CRITERIA

Short-term:
- Begins to deal with incident of sexual abuse by openly discussing event by second session.
- Verbalizes understanding of male sexual feelings and discusses concerns with her mate within 3 sessions.
- Demonstrates improved communication/ relationship skills by sixth session.

Long-term:
- Verbalizes acceptance of self as an adequate sexual woman by discharge from therapy.

Actions/Interventions	Rationale
Encourage open discussion of concerns and expression of feelings. Assist with problem solving.	Promotes thinking about causes/results of behaviors and suggests new ways to resolve problems.
Discuss incident of sexual abuse in childhood and identify how it affects current	Awareness of what has occurred and how it has affected her life will allow for understanding of

relationship.

own responses/behavior and assist in making desired changes in how she relates to the men in her life.

Evaluate knowledge base and provide sex information/education as indicated.

Accurate knowledge will help understanding and promote effective decision making about relationships.

Explore relationship with current mate, discussing interactions that lead to fighting and distancing.

Provides opportunity for identification of problem areas and assists with problem solving.

Encourage use of I-messages and other assertiveness skills to deal with put-downs of mate.

Use of clear communication skills enhances resolution of problems/enhances self-esteem and promotes sense of control over self/situation.

Discuss ways in which she can learn to take care of herself (i.e., making time for own pleasure, making own choices).

Acknowledges herself as a worthwhile person, enhancing her self-esteem.

Determine relationship with

Promotes awareness of how her behavior

Actions/Interventions	Rationale
daughter. Discuss effective parenting skills she can use, (e.g., Active-listening and problem solving).	provides a role model for her daughter and ways in which she can establish a relationship in which she becomes a more positive influence.
Recommend attendance at group therapy for sexual abuse and assertiveness training classes.	Sharing with others who have similar experiences helps client to gain insight and promotes behavioral change.

HOME HEALTH/ REHABILITATION PATIENT SITUATION: TRAUMA

B.R., a 37-year-old iron worker, was injured on 11/6 when a large steel girder fell 10 feet from a crane, pinning him to the ground. He was admitted to the hospital on that date with fractured ribs (left 9, 10, and 11), a fractured pelvis (left ileum), internal injuries (requiring splenectomy), soft-tissue trauma, and significant blood loss (see Critical Care Situation: Multiple Trauma, p. 109).

The ruptured spleen and a large hematoma of the left thigh created an initial anemia (sequestration of blood) for which transfusions were given. Additionally, circulation, sensation, and function of the left leg were impaired, causing swelling, pain, and potentiating risk of thrombophlebitis/emboli.

His postoperative course was uneventful as related to healing of the abdominal incision and restoration of gastrointestinal function. However, he did develop respiratory complications (atelectasis and pneumonia) related to rib fractures and immobility.

Soft-tissue injuries to B.R.'s chest and left shoulder resulted in multiple ecchymotic areas that are clearing slowly. He wears a rib belt to support his fractured ribs. The linear fracture of the pelvis is painful, but does not prevent B.R. from progressive activity. It has, however, affected his ability to sit comfortably and to change position readily, and it increases the risk of falls (balance problem). He has started on a physical therapy program to instruct him in the use of a walker with progression to crutches when able. Discharge planning includes referral to rehabilitation services for evaluation of home-care needs and possible therapy.

Ongoing and potential long-term problems are related to the length of time required for the healing of fractures and soft-tissue injury.

DISCHARGE PHYSICIAN ORDERS

Make home visit to assess needs of environment.
Physical therapy three times per week for continuation of current program.
Enteric-coated ASA 10 gr daily.
Darvocet-N 100 ii PO q 4 to 6 hr for pain.

DISCHARGE CONSIDERATIONS

Date re-evaluated: 11/19
Anticipated discharge: 11/21
Resources: Person: Wife, mother, 3 brothers and sisters-in-law; P.W., RN, medical care coordinator.
Financial: Workmen's Compensation (short- and long-term disability), sick leave and some savings available to meet future needs as required.
Anticipated areas requiring assistance:

1. Physical layout of home: To sleep in downstairs guest bedroom at this time.
2. Ambulation: Walker/crutches rented from Home Care Needs.
3. Self care: Grab bars to be installed in first floor bathroom tub and toilet area (brother R.R.). Bath chair rented from Home Care Needs.
4. Nutrition: Lunch to be prepared by mother/sisters-in-law.
5. Rehabilitation program: Physical therapy three times per week in hospital.
6. Transportation: Sisters-in-law will rotate for therapy and medical follow-up.

HOME HEALTH/ REHABILITATION CARE PLAN: TRAUMA

PATIENT PROBLEM STATEMENT/ FOCUS (NURSING DIAGNOSIS)

Mobility, impaired, physical related to neuromuscular skeletal impairment, pain/discomfort, decreased muscle strength/control, or decreased strength and endurance as evidenced by weakness, limited range of motion, lack of coordination, reluctance to attempt movement, difficulty moving purposefully within physical environment.

PATIENT OUTCOMES/ EVALUATION CRITERIA

- Demonstrates stepped improvement in range of motion, strength, and function of L arm/leg on a weekly basis.
- Performs self-care activities within level of own ability showing progressive movement weekly toward independence.
- Uses personal/community resources to provide assistance appropriately (ongoing).

Actions/Interventions	Rationale
Assess functional ability (NANDA scale 0–4) and reevaluate weekly three times, then as indicated.	Identifies areas of need allowing for individualized interventions.
Identify barriers to participation in regimen.	Interference can occur because of numerous factors

Actions/Interventions	Rationale
	(e.g., lack of information, continuing pain and fatigue, post-trauma stress response).
Identify activities B.R. can perform independently and those requiring assistance.	On initial evaluation, patient can feed self, shave, and brush hair and teeth. He requires assistance with dressing, shower and shampoo, and transfer from bed to chair and from chair to walker.
Involve B.R. and family caregiver members in problem-solving solutions to individual needs (e.g., transportation to health-care appointments, assuming lawn-care activities, shared schedule for diversional visits/ outings as able).	Provides options, allows members choices for maximal participation with minimal intrusion into own life/responsibilities.
Arrange for necessary assistive devices through Home Care Needs. Provide telephone contact	Equipment and services can be supplied. Patient/ wife will benefit from instruction and

numbers.	support, especially in emergency situations.
Help B.R./wife set weekly goals. Demonstrate use of progress flow sheets if they deem them useful.	Provides positive objective feedback for efforts, progress made, (e.g., walked 50 feet to the mailbox unassisted).
Allow sufficient time for B.R. to complete tasks.	Decreases discouragement and improves general strength and self-reliance.
Recommend periods of activity balanced with rest.	Reduces fatigue and muscle tension to improve general mobility.
Monitor circulation/ sensation in left foot and left hand, noting edema, temperature, or color changes. Instruct B.R. to report changes in sensation or movement (e.g., tingling, burning pain, pain in calf, and weakness).	Thigh hematoma may take several weeks to completely resolve (sequestered a unit of blood following injury) and may continue to cause problems associated with compression of nerves, ischemia, and/or altered clotting mechanisms.
Teach B.R./wife how to support affected body parts in all positions (e.g.,	Promotes comfort and reduces risk of pressure or stretch injuries to nerves.

Actions/Interventions	Rationale
when sitting, lying, and standing).	
Recommend use of lounge chair for sitting.	Fractured pelvis may require up to 6 weeks to heal. Lounge chair allows for more even distribution of weight with elevation of feet/legs to promote venous return.
Progressively increase exercise program as tolerated.	Improves general strength and will help restore normal function and mobility as healing occurs.
Evaluate degree of pain using 1–10 scale each time pain is discussed.	Establishes a consistent way to identify and discuss current level of pain, changes in pain, and effectiveness of comfort measures and/or medication.
Encourage use of pain medication before activity/exercise as indicated.	Reduces muscle spasm, enhancing participation in activity program.
Observe emotional/behavioral	Helps identify strengths and

responses to problems of immobility.

deficits (needed for safety reinforcement, encouragement, and goal achievement). Also helps to identify psychologic impact of pain and coping methods.

Encourage expression of feelings and discuss concerns.

Promotes awareness of feelings and provides opportunity to look at options for coping. Also reduces anxiety and tension associated with trauma and early recuperative period.

Note movement when patient is unaware of observation. Discuss discrepancies, if present, in a nonjudgmental manner.

Helps B.R. to identify difficulties that may be based on fear rather than physical inability to move.

PATIENT PROBLEM STATEMENT/ FOCUS (NURSING DIAGNOSIS)

Knowledge deficit [learning need] related to lack of exposure to information, misinterpretation, unfamiliarity with information resources as evidenced by request for information, statement of misconception, and verbalization of problem.

DESIRED PATIENT OUTCOMES/ EVALUATION CRITERIA

- Verbalizes understanding of relationship of injuries and associated complications to rehabilitation needs by 11/23.
- Correctly performs necessary procedures and explains reasons for actions by 11/23.
- Continues cessation of smoking with participation in treatment program (ongoing).

Actions/Interventions	Rationale
Review pathology, prognosis, and future expectations.	Provides knowledge base on which patient can make informed choices.
Include wife in teaching sessions.	Wife will be the coordinator of care at home and needs information and support.
Determine most urgent need from patient's, significant others', and nurse's viewpoint.	Helps to focus teaching and addresses priorities as identified.
Observe B.R.'s adherence to safety factors when ambulating.	Weakness and feeling of unbalance caused by fractured pelvis and pain may cause him to stagger. Psychologic effects of pain may also be noted.

Reinforce physical therapist's teaching regarding proper method of transfers, use of walker for ambulation, shower chair, and so forth.	Promotes independence and rapid learning, enhancing safe movement.
Encourage continuation of exercise/physical therapy program (e.g., feet/ankle exercises while at rest, passive ROM exercise of L shoulder by wife).	Physical therapy appointments are three times per week. Continued participation promotes healing of fractures, prevents muscle atrophy, reduces muscle spasm, and promotes earlier return to desired activity level.
Identify signs/symptoms requiring medical evaluation (e.g., severe pain, fever/chills, changes in sensation, etc.).	Prompt intervention may reduce severity of complications that could occur. Late complications would likely be the result of the large hematoma of the leg and/or fractures (e.g., emboli).
Review importance of well-balanced diet and increased fluids.	Although more calories are needed to facilitate healing, weight gain is not desirable at this time because of risk of increased pain

Actions/Interventions	Rationale
	and mobility problems. Increasing fluids reduces constipation and flushes toxins from the body.
Recognize level of achievement and discuss time factors to achieve short-term and long-term goals.	Understanding present and future expectations may improve patient's self-esteem and hope for timely recovery.
Provide written information/guidelines.	Helpful for patient/wife to refer to as necessary.
Provide phone number of contact person(s).	To answer questions/make referrals after discharge.
Identify/refer to community resources as appropriate (e.g., vocational rehabilitation, social services, employer, smoking support group [if necessary]).	May require additional information and support during the recovery period to meet financial responsibilities and eventually return to gainful employment.
Review medication instructions (written and verbal)	Enhances cooperation with drug regimen, maximizing

regarding dosage, schedule, purpose/action of drugs, and expected and reportable side effects.	therapeutic effects and minimizing potential problems.
Recommend avoidance of crowds/persons with infectious diseases.	Resistance is lower/immune system stressed, increasing risk of acquired illness.
Discuss importance of clinical follow-up appointments.	Patient is recovering from major abdominal surgery as well as multiple trauma and needs ongoing supervision to prevent complications from developing.

PATIENT PROBLEM STATEMENT/ FOCUS (NURSING DIAGNOSIS)

Post-trauma, response, potential related to sudden traumatic accident.

PATIENT OUTCOMES/ EVALUATION CRITERIA

- Reports improvement in sleep/rest pattern within 2 weeks.
- Verbalizes reduced anxiety/fear when memories occur (ongoing).
- Demonstrates ability to deal with emotional reactions in an individual, appropriate manner (ongoing).

Actions/Interventions	Rationale
Identify whether incident has reactivated pre-existing or coexisting situations, job/personal difficulties.	These factors can add to the anxiety and concern that accompany current trauma, resulting in an increased possibility of development of post-trauma response.
Note withdrawn behavior and use of denial.	Indicators that B.R. is having problem adjusting to accident and lengthy convalescence.
Encourage discussion of the accident and verbalization of feelings and concerns about the future.	Talking about the accident is an important step toward recovery; awareness and acceptance of accompanying feelings promote resolution.
Discuss probability of emotional reactions (e.g., withdrawal, angry outbursts, tears). Encourage development of effective coping skills.	Understanding that these are common reactions and usually subside with the passage of time can help the patient to accept and deal with these feelings.
Discuss ways to	Trauma patients

reduce sleep disturbances (e.g., use of pain medication at bedtime, padding and positioning with pillows, etc.). Identify and teach skills of visual imagery, relaxation, and use of breathing exercises.

frequently have difficulty with falling asleep and waking up in pain. Use of relaxation and imagery techniques can reduce tension and assist patient to rest/sleep appropriately.

Address possibility of dreams and nightmares.

Often occurs in acute post-trauma stage and usually resolves in a few days or weeks.

Discuss changes in lifestyle that may be anticipated.

Will help B.R. look at possibilities and how they can contribute to recovery.

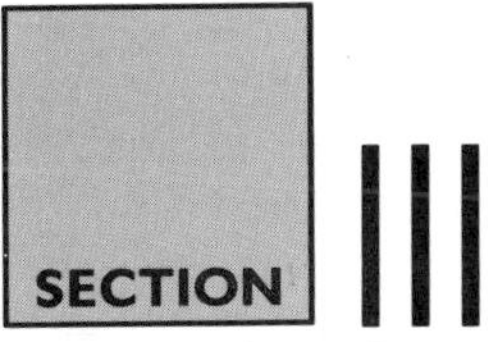

SECTION III

300 DISORDERS/ HEALTH PROBLEMS WITH ASSOCIATED NURSING DIAGNOSES

Section III presents 300 disorders/health problems, reflecting all specialty areas, with associated nursing diagnoses. The health problems with their associated nursing diagnoses are written as patient problem statements and include "related to" and "evidenced by" statements.

The section will facilitate and validate the assessment and diagnosis steps of the nursing process. Because the nursing process is perpetual and ongoing, other nursing diagnoses may be appropriate based on changing individual situations. Therefore, the nurse must continually assess, identify, and validate new problems and evaluate subsequent care. Once appropriate nursing diagnoses have been selected, the reader is encouaged to refer to **Nurse's Pocket Guide:*

---

*Specific focus on assessment data, desired patient outcomes/evaluation criteria, and general interventions for each NANDA nursing diagnosis can be found in *Nurse's Pocket Guide: Nursing Diagnoses with Interventions*, ed 2, F.A. Davis, 1988. Revised reprint 1989.

Nursing Diagnoses with Interventions to assist in identifying other nursing diagnoses based on the changing needs of the patient. *Nurse's Pocket Guide* will enable you to construct and tailor a care plan by means of the book's generalized interventions and desired patient outcomes/evaluation criteria for each NANDA diagnosis. Although each of the books can be used alone, when used together, they provide the basic tools necessary to construct care plans for every patient situation in all nursing specialty areas.

To facilitate access to the disorders and nursing diagnoses, the disorders have been listed alphabetically and coded to identify nursing specialty areas.

Key: MS: Medical-Surgical CH: Community
PED: Pediatric OB: Obstetrical
GYN: Gynecologic PSY: Psychiatric

(Note: Information that appears in brackets has been added by the authors to clarify and enhance the use of nursing diagnosis). The phrases "may be related to" and "possibly evidenced by" in the patient problem statements are used to indicate that the information should be selected to reflect an individual patient/situation. Knowledge deficit, although implied in each disorder/health problem, has been included only in some conditions to provide examples.

■ A

ABORTION, SPONTANEOUS OB

Fluid volume deficit (2) [active loss] may be related to excessive blood loss possibly evidenced by hypotension, decreased pulse volume and pressure, delayed capillary refill, or changes in sensorium

Tissue perfusion, altered, (specify) may be related to hypovolemia, possibly evidenced by: *peripheral:* hypotension, cool/pale skin, diminished pulses; *cerebral:* changes in sensorium; *renal:* decreased urinary output.

Anxiety (specify level) may be related to changes in health status of fetus/self, threat of death possibly evidenced by restlessness, tremors, facial tension, focus on self, or feeling of uncertainty.

*Infection, potential for** may be related to altered

---

*Note: A potential diagnosis is not evidenced by signs and symptoms as the problem has not occurred and nursing interventions are directed at prevention.

myometrial integrity at site of placental attachment, surgically traumatized tissues, and/or decreased hemoglobin.

Knowledge deficit [learning need] may be related to lack of familiarity with new self/health-care needs, sources for support possibly evidenced by requests for information, statement of concern/misconceptions.

Grieving [expected] may be related to perinatal loss possibly evidenced by crying, expressions of sorrow, or changes in eating habits/sleep pattern.

ABRUPTIO PLACENTA — OB

Fluid volume deficit (2) [active loss] may be related to excessive blood loss possibly evidenced by hypotension, decreased pulse volume and pressure, delayed capillary refill, or changes in sensorium.

Anxiety (specify level) may be related to threat of death of fetus and/or self possibly evidenced by focus on self, facial tension, restlessness, feelings of uncertainty, or expressions of concern.

Pain may be related to collection of blood between uterine wall and placenta possibly evidenced by verbal complaints, abdominal guarding, muscle tension, or alterations in vital signs.

Gas exchange, impaired, fetal may be related to altered utero-placental oxygen transfer possibly evidenced by alterations in fetal heart rate and movement.

ABSCESS, BRAIN (ACUTE) — MS

Pain may be related to inflammation, edema of tissues possibly evidenced by complaints of headache, restlessness, irritability, and moaning.

*Body temperature, altered, potential** may be related to inflammatory process/hypermetabolic state and dehydration.

---

*See footnote on following page.

Thought processes, altered may be related to physiologic changes (e.g., cerebral edema/altered perfusion, fever) possibly evidenced by inability to follow commands, altered attention span, or disorientation.

*Suffocation/Trauma, potential for** may be related to development of clonic/tonic muscle activity and changes in consciousness (seizure activity).

ACHALASIA

MS

Nutrition, altered: Less than body requirements may be related to inability and/or reluctance to ingest adequate nutrients to meet metabolic demands possibly evidenced by reported/observed inadequate intake, weight loss, pale conjunctiva, and mucous membranes.

Pain may be related to spasm of the lower esophageal sphincter possibly evidenced by complaints of substernal pressure, recurrent heartburn, or gastric fullness (gas pains).

Anxiety (specify level)/Fear may be related to recurrent pain, choking sensation, altered health status possibly evidenced by verbalization of distress, apprehension, restlessness, or insomnia.

*Aspiration, potential for** may be related to regurgitation/spillover of esophageal contents.

CH

Knowledge deficit [learning need] may be related to lack of familiarity with pathology and treatment of condition possibly evidenced by requests for information, statement of concern, or development of preventable complications.

---

*Note: A potential diagnosis is not evidenced by signs and symptoms as the problem has not occurred and nursing interventions are directed at prevention.

Swallowing, impaired may be related to neuromuscular impairment possibly evidenced by observed evidence of difficulty swallowing, or regurgitation.

ACIDOSIS, METABOLIC MS

(Refer to Diabetic Ketoacidosis)

ADDISON'S DISEASE MS

Fluid volume deficit, (1) [regulatory failure] may be related to vomiting, diarrhea, increased renal losses possibly evidenced by delayed capillary refill, poor skin turgor, dry mucous membranes, or complaints of thirst.

Cardiac output, decreased may be related to hypovolemia and altered electrical conduction/dysrthymias and/or diminished cardiac muscle mass possibly evidenced by alterations in vital signs, changes in mentation, and irregular pulse or pulse deficit.

Fatigue may be related to decreased metabolic energy production, altered body chemistry (fluid, electrolyte, and glucose imbalance) possibly evidenced by unremitting/overwhelming lack of energy, inability to maintain usual routines, decreased performance, impaired ability to concentrate, lethargy, and disinterest in surroundings.

Body image disturbance may be related to changes in skin pigmentation, mucous membranes, loss of axillary/pubic hair possibly evidenced by verbalization of negative feelings about body and decreased social involvement.

*Mobility, impaired, physical, potential** may be

---

*Note: A potential diagnosis is not evidenced by signs and symptoms as the problem has not occurred and nursing interventions are directed at prevention.

related to neuromuscular impairment (muscle wasting/weakness) and dizziness/syncope.

CH

Nutrition, altered: Less than body requirements may be related to glucocorticoid deficiency; abnormal fat, protein, and carbohydrate metabolism, nausea, vomiting, anorexia possibly evidenced by weight loss, muscle wasting, abdominal cramps, diarrhea, and severe hypoglycemia.

*Home maintenance management, impaired, potential** may be related to effects of disease process, impaired cognitive functioning, and inadequate support systems.

ADENOIDECTOMY — PED

Anxiety (specify level)/Fear may be related to separation from supportive others, unfamiliar surroundings, and perceived threat of death possibly evidenced by crying, apprehension, trembling, and sympathetic stimulation (pupil dilation, increased heart rate).

*Airway clearance, ineffective, potential** may be related to sedation, collection of secretions/blood in oropharynx, and vomiting.

*Fluid volume deficit, potential** may be related to operative trauma to highly vascular site resulting in hemorrhage.

Pain may be related to physical trauma to oronasopharynx, presence of packing possibly evidenced by restlessness, crying, and facial mask of pain.

---

*Note: A potential diagnosis is not evidenced by signs and symptoms as the problem has not occurred and nursing interventions are directed at prevention.

ADRENALECTOMY MS

Tissue perfusion, altered, (specify) may be related to hypovolemia and vascular pooling (vasodilation) possibly evidenced by diminished pulses, pallor/cyanosis, hypotension, and changes in mentation.

Skin integrity, impaired related to presence of surgical incision evidenced by disruption of skin surface and mechanical closure (sutures/staples).

Knowledge deficit [learning need] may be related to unfamiliarity with long-term therapy requirements possibly evidenced by request for information and statement of concern/misconception.

ADULT RESPIRATORY DISTRESS SYNDROME MS

Airway Clearance, ineffective may be related to decreased ciliary action, increased amount and viscosity of secretions, and collapse of small airways possibly evidenced by presence of rhonchi/rales, gurgling respirations and recurrent cough.

Gas exchange, impaired may be related to changes in pulmonary capillary permeability with edema formation, alveolar collapse with intrapulmonary shunting possibly evidenced by tachypnea, use of accessory muscles, retractions, cyanosis, and changes in mentation.

*Fluid volume, deficit, potential** may be related to active loss from diuretic use, and restricted intake.

*Fluid volume, excess, potential** may be related to excessive sodium/fluid retention or administration.

*Cardiac output, decreased, potential** may be related to alteration in pre-load (hypovolemia, vascu-

---

*Note: A potential diagnosis is not evidenced by signs and symptoms as the problem has not occurred and nursing interventions are directed at prevention.

lar pooling, diuretic therapy, and increased intrathoracic pressure/use of PEEP).

Anxiety (specify level)/Fear may be related to situational crisis, change in health status/threat of death possibly evidenced by increased tension, apprehension, restlessness, sympathetic stimulation, and focus on self.

AFFECTIVE DISORDER — PSY

(Refer to Bipolar Disorders and Depressive Disorders, Major)

AIDS (ACQUIRED IMMUNE DEFICIENCY SYNDROME) — MS

*Infection, potential for,** progression to sepsis/overgrowth may be related to suppressed inflammatory response and immunosuppression in combination with inadequate primary defenses and malnutrition.

*Fluid volume deficit, potential** may be related to excessive losses: copious diarrhea, profuse sweating, vomiting, hypermetabolic state, and fever; restricted intake: nausea and anorexia; lethargy.

*Injury, potential for, altered clotting factors** may be related to decreased vitamin K absorption, alteration in hepatic function, presence of autoimmune antiplatelet antibodies, malignancies (Kaposi's sarcoma), and circulating endotoxins (sepsis).

Pain may be related to tissue inflammation/destruction: infections, internal/external cutaneous lesions, rectal excoriation, malignancies, necrosis; myalgias and arthralgias, abdominal cramping possibly evidenced by complaints of pain, self-focusing/narrowed focus, alteration in muscle tone,

---

*Note: A potential diagnosis is not evidenced by signs and symptoms as the problem has not occurred and nursing interventions are directed at prevention.

guarding behaviors, autonomic responses, and restlessness.

Skin integrity, impaired may be related to immunologic deficit (AIDS-related dermatitis, bacterial/fungal infections, opportunistic disease processes/Kaposi's sarcoma), decreased level of activity, altered sensation, skeletal prominence, altered metabolic state possibly evidenced by skin lesions; ulcerations; decubitus ulcer formation.

CH

Fatigue may be related to decreased metabolic energy production, increased energy requirements (hypermetabolic state), overwhelming psychologic/emotional demands, altered body chemistry, (side effects of medication, chemotherapy) possibly evidenced by unremitting/overwhelming lack of energy, inability to maintain usual routines, decreased performance; impaired ability to concentrate, lethargy/listlessness, and disinterest in surroundings.

Nutrition, altered: Less than body requirements may be related to inability to ingest, digest, and/or absorb nutrients; nausea/vomiting, hyperactive gag reflex, intestinal disturbances, increased metabolic activity/nutritional needs (fever, infection) possibly evidenced by weight loss, decreased subcutaneous fat/muscle mass, lack of interest in food/aversion to eating, altered taste sensation, abdominal cramping, hyperactive bowel sounds, diarrhea, sore and inflamed buccal cavity.

*Health maintenance, altered, potential** may be related to lack of material resources, impaired adjustment, and inadequate support systems.

---

*Note: A potential diagnosis is not evidenced by signs and symptoms as the problem has not occurred and nursing interventions are directed at prevention.

*Home maintenance management, impaired, potential** may be related to effects of disease process, insufficient finances, and inadequate support systems.

PSY

Social isolation may be related to alterations in physical appearance, state of wellness, phobic fear of others (transmission of disease) possibly evidenced by expressed feelings of rejection, absence of supportive significant others, and withdrawal from usual activities.

Thought processes, altered may be related to physiologic changes, for example, hypoxemia, CNS infection by HIV, brain malignancies, and/or disseminated systemic opportunistic infection; alteration of drug metabolism/excretion, accumulation of toxic elements (renal failure, severe electrolyte imbalance, hepatic insufficiency) possibly evidenced by altered attention span, distractibility, memory deficit, disorientation, cognitive dissonance, delusional thinking, sleep disturbances, impaired ability to make decisions/problem solve, inability to follow complex commands/mental tasks, and loss of impulse control.

Powerlessness may be related to confirmed diagnosis of a terminal disease, incomplete grieving process, social ramifications of AIDS, alteration in body image, changes in desired lifestyle; progression of disease process possibly evidenced by feelings of loss of control over own life, depression over physical deterioration that occurs despite patient compliance with regimen, anger, apathy, with-

---

*Note: A potential diagnosis is not evidenced by signs and symptoms as the problem has not occurred and nursing interventions are directed at prevention.

drawal, passivity, dependence on others for care/decision making, resentment, and guilt.

ALDOSTERONISM, PRIMARY MS

Fluid volume deficit, (1) [regulatory failure] may be related to increased urinary losses possibly evidenced by dry mucous membranes, poor skin turgor, dilute urine, excessive thirst, weight loss.

Mobility impaired, physical may be related to neuromuscular impairment, weakness, and pain possibly evidenced by impaired coordination, decreased muscle strength, paralysis, and positive Chvostek's and Trousseau's signs.

*Cardiac output, decreased, potential** may be related to hypovolemia and altered electrical conduction/dysrhythmias.

ALZHEIMER'S DISEASE CH/PSY

*Trauma, potential for** may be related to inability to recognize/identify danger in environment, disorientation, confusion, impaired judgment, weakness, and muscular incoordination.

Thought processes, altered may be related to physiologic changes (neuronal degeneration), sleep deprivation possibly evidenced by memory deficit, impaired ability to make decisions/problem solve, distractibility, disorientation.

Sensory-perceptual, alterations (specify) may be related to neurologic deficit (irreversible neuronal degeneration, sleep deprivation), environmental factors (socially restricted environment/homebound or institutionalization) possibly evidenced by memory loss, changes in usual response to stimuli,

---

*Note: A potential diagnosis is not evidenced by signs and symptoms as the problem has not occurred and nursing interventions are directed at prevention.

spatial disorientation, confusion, exaggerated emotional responses, anxiety, paranoia, and hallucinations, inability to tell position of body parts, and diminished/altered sense of taste.

Self-care deficit (specify) may be related to perceptual/cognitive impairment, unstable gait possibly evidenced by forgetfulness, disheveled appearance, body odor, incontinence, and decreased dietary intake.

Sleep pattern disturbance may be related to disorientation (day/night reversal), irritability, poor judgment potentiated by neurologic impairment possibly evidenced by wakefulness and increased aimless wandering, inability to identify need/time for sleeping.

Fear may be related to decreased ability in function, public disclosure of disabilities, progressive mental/physical deterioration possibly evidenced by social isolation, aggressive behavior, apprehension, irritability, defensiveness, and suspiciousness.

Grieving, anticipatory may be related to perceived potential loss of self possibly evidenced by expressions of sorrow and anger, altered sleep and/or eating patterns, changes in activity level, and libido.

Family coping, ineffective, compromised may be related to family disorganization, role changes, long-term illness exhausting supportive/financial capabilities of family member(s) possibly evidenced by verbalizations of frustrations in dealing with day-to-day care, expressed anger/guilt directed toward patient, and withdrawal from interaction with patient.

Home maintenance management, impaired may be related to progressive impaired cognitive functioning, insufficient family organization or planning, unfamiliarity with resources, inadequate support systems possibly evidenced by household members expressing difficulty/requesting help in maintaining home in comfortable fashion, lack of necessary equipment or aids to care for patient, overtaxed family members, and disorderly surroundings.

Health maintenance, altered may be related to deterioration affecting ability in all areas, cognitive impairment, ineffective individual/family coping, dysfunctional grieving possibly evidenced by reported or observed inability to take responsibility for meeting basic health practices, reported or observed lack of equipment/financial or other resources, and reported or observed impairment of personal support system.

AMPUTATION MS

Body image disturbance may be related to loss of a body part possibly evidenced by verbalization of feelings of powerlessness, grief, preoccupation with loss, and unwillingness to look at/touch stump.

*Fluid volume, deficit, potential** may be related to vascular loss (hemorrhage).

Pain may be related to tissue trauma, severed nerves possibly evidenced by complaints of incisional/phantom pain, guarding behavior, and narrowed focus.

Mobility, impaired physical may be related to loss of limb, altered sense of balance possibly evidenced by impaired coordination, unsteady gait, and difficulty/inability to ambulate.

AMYOTROPHIC LATERAL SCLEROSIS MS

Mobility, impaired physical may be related to muscle wasting/weakness possibly evidenced by

---

*Note: A potential diagnosis is not evidenced by signs and symptoms as the problem has not occurred and nursing interventions are directed at prevention.

impaired coordination, limited range of motion, and impaired purposeful movement.

Breathing pattern, ineffective may be related to neuromuscular impairment, decreased energy, fatigue, tracheobronchial obstruction possibly evidenced by shortness of breath, fremitus, respiratory depth changes, and reduced vital capacity.

Body image disturbance may be related to prolonged, debilitating illness with loss of ability to control body possibly evidenced by verbalization of negative feelings about body, helplessness, observed decrease in social involvement.

Swallowing, impaired may be related to muscle wasting and fatigue possibly evidenced by recurrent coughing/choking and evidence of aspiration.

Powerlessness may be related to debilitating nature of illness, lack of control over outcome possibly evidenced by expressions of frustration about inability to care for self and depression over physical deterioration.

CH

Communication, impaired, verbal may be related to physical barrier (neuromuscular impairment) possibly evidenced by impaired articulation, inability to speak in sentences, and use of nonverbal cues (changes in facial expression).

Self-care deficit may be related to neuromuscular impairment, decreased strength/endurance, depression possibly evidenced by inability to perform tasks satisfactorily, disheveled appearance, body odor, and decreased dietary intake.

Grieving, anticipatory may be related to perceived potential loss of self, physio-psychosocial well-being possibly evidenced by sorrow, choked feelings, expression of distress, changes in eating habits/sleeping patterns, and altered libido.

Home maintenance management, impaired may be related to effects of disease, inadequate support systems, change in financial status possibly evidenced by lack of necessary equipment or aids, overtaxed family members.

ANEMIA CH

Activity intolerance may be related to imbalance between oxygen supply and demand possibly evidenced by reports of fatigue and weakness, abnormal heart rate with activity, and exertional dyspnea.

Knowledge deficit [learning need] may be related to inadequate understanding or misinterpretation of dietary/physiologic needs possibly evidenced by inadequate dietary intake, request for information, and development of preventable complications.

ANEMIA: SICKLE CELL MS

Gas exchange, impaired may be related to altered oxygen-carrying capacity of blood possibly evidenced by signs of hypoxia, changes in mentation, and restlessness.

Pain may be related to localized vascular stasis and occlusion possibly evidenced by complaints of migratory joint and/or abdominal/back pain, and guarding/distraction behaviors (moaning, crying, restlessness).

Tissue perfusion, altered, (specify) may be related to stasis, occlusion of arterial/venous blood flow possibly evidenced by signs and symptoms dependent on system involved, for example: *renal:* decreased specific gravity and pale urine in face of dehydration; *cerebral:* paralysis and decreased visual acuity; *peripheral:* distal ischemia and tissue infarctions.

Knowledge deficit [learning need] may be related to lack of exposure/recall regarding disease process, genetic factors, prognosis and treatment needs, misinterpretation of information possibly evidenced by questions, statement of concern/misconceptions, exacerbation of condition, inadequate follow-through of therapy instructions, and development of preventable complications.

PED

Growth and development, altered may be related to effects of physical condition possibly evidenced by altered physical growth and delay/difficulty performing skills typical of age group.

Family coping, ineffective, compromised may be related to chronic nature of disease/disability, parenteral supervision, and lifestyle restrictions possibly evidenced by protective behavior disproportionate to patient's ability or need for autonomy.

ANGINA PECTORIS MS

Pain may be related to ischemia of cardiac muscle possibly evidenced by complaints of pain, narrowed focus, distraction behaviors (restlessness, moaning), and automatic responses (diaphoresis, elevation of vital signs).

Cardiac output, decreased may be related to inotropic changes (transient/prolonged myocardial ischemia, effects of medications), alterations in rate/rhythm and electrical conduction possibly evidenced by changes in hemodynamic readings, dyspnea, restlessness, decreased tolerance for activity, fatigue, diminished peripheral pulses, cool/pale skin, changes in mental status, and continued chest pain.

Anxiety (specify level) may be related to change in health status and/or threat of death possibly evidenced by verbalized apprehension, facial tension, extraneous movements, and focus on self.

Activity intolerance may be related to imbalance between oxygen supply and demand possibly evidenced by exertional dypspnea, abnormal pulse/blood pressure response to activity, and ECG changes.

CH

Knowledge deficit [learning need] may be related to lack of exposure, inaccurate/misinterpretation of information regarding disease process, prognosis and treatment needs possibly evidenced by questions, request for information, statement of concern, and inaccurate follow-through of instructions.

*Adjustment, impaired, potential** may be related to condition requiring long-term therapy/change in lifestyle, assault to self-esteem, and altered locus of control.

ANOREXIA NERVOSA — MS/PSY

Nutrition, altered: Less than body requirements may be related to psychologic restrictions of food intake and/or excessive activity possibly evidenced by weight loss, denial of hunger, and unusual hoarding or handling of food.

*Fluid volume deficit, potential** may be related to inadequate intake of food and liquids, consistent self-induced vomiting, and laxative/diuretic use.

Body image disturbance may be related to altered perception of body possibly evidenced by negative feelings about body, preoccupation with perceived image of self as fat, and change in social involvement.

Coping ineffective, individual may be related to maturational crisis and attempt to control environment, possibly evidenced by verbalization of poor self-esteem and difficulty meeting role expectations, and poor problem-solving capabilities.

Family coping, ineffective, disabling may be related to ambivalent family relationships and ways of transacting issues of control possibly evidenced by

---

*Note: A potential diagnosis is not evidenced by signs and symptoms as the problem has not occurred and nursing interventions are directed at prevention.

enmeshed family with lack of separation of individual members who may speak for one another.

ANXIETY DISORDERS

(DEPENDENT ON DEGREE) **PSY**

Anxiety (specify level)/Powerlessness may be related to real or perceived threat to physical integrity or self-concept (may or may not be able to identify the threat), unconscious conflict about essential values/beliefs and goals of life, unmet needs, positive or negative self-talk possibly evidenced by persistent feelings of apprehension and uneasiness, a general anxious feeling that patient has difficulty alleviating, sympathetic stimulation, extraneous movements (foot shuffling, hand/arm fidgeting, rocking movements, restlessness), poor eye contact, focus on self, impaired functioning, and free-floating anxiety.

Sleep pattern disturbance may be related to psychologic stress, repetitive thoughts possibly evidenced by reports of difficulty in falling asleep/awakening earlier or later than desired, complaints of not feeling rested, dark circles under eyes, and frequent yawning.

Coping, ineffective, individual may be related to unrealistic perceptions and inadequate coping methods possibly evidenced by verbalization of inability to cope/problem solve, excessive compulsive behaviors (e.g., smoking, drinking), and emotional tension.

Fear may be related to phobic stimulus possibly evidenced by response ranging from apprehension to panic, fight or flight response, and sympathetic stimulation (pupil dilation, increased heart rate).

Social interaction, impaired may be related to low self-esteem and misinterpretation of internal/external stimuli possibly evidenced by discomfort in social situations and withdrawal from or reported change in pattern of interactions.

AORTIC STENOSIS MS

Cardiac output, decreased may be related to structural changes of heart valve possibly evidenced by fatigue, dyspnea, altered vital signs, and syncope.

Activity intolerance may be related to imbalance between oxygen supply and demand possibly evidenced by exertional dyspnea, reported fatigue/weakness, and ECG changes/dysrhythmias.

Pain may be related to ischemia of cardiac muscle possibly evidenced by verbal complaints of pain, facial grimacing, narrowed focus, and autonomic responses (alterations in vital signs).

APPENDICITIS MS

Pain may be related to inflammation possibly evidenced by complaints of pain, guarding behavior, narrowed focus, and automatic responses (diaphoresis, changes in vital signs).

*Fluid volume, deficit, potential** may be related to nausea, vomiting, and anorexia.

*Infection, potential for** may be related to release of pathogenic organisms into peritoneal cavity.

ARRHYTHMIA, CARDIAC MS/CH

(Refer to Dysrhythmias)

ARTHRITIS, JUVENILE RHEUMATOID PED/CH

(Refer Also to Arthritis, Rheumatoid)

Growth and development, altered may be related to effects of physical disability and required therapy possibly evidenced by lack of/delayed physical growth appropriate for age.

---

*Note: A potential diagnosis is not evidenced by signs and symptoms as the problem has not occurred and nursing interventions are directed at prevention.

*Social isolation, potential** may be related to delay in accomplishing developmental task, altered state of wellness, and changes in physical appearance.

ARTHRITIS, RHEUMATOID CH

Pain, chronic may be related to joint/muscle inflammation, degeneration, deformity possibly evidenced by complaints of pain, narrowed focus, guarded movement, and physical and social withdrawal.

Mobility, impaired physical may be related to musculoskeletal impairment and pain possibly evidenced by limited range of motion, reluctance to attempt movement, and decreased muscle strength.

Self-care deficit (specify) may be related to decreased strength/range of motion, pain possibly evidenced by reported difficulties in performing tasks.

Body image disturbance may be related to change in body structure/function possibly evidenced by negative feelings about body, feelings of helplessness, and preoccupation with change or loss.

ARTHROPLASTY MS

*Infection, potential for** may be related to breach of primary defenses by surgical incision, stasis of body fluids at operative site, and altered inflammatory response.

*Fluid volume deficit, potential** may be related to excessive vascular loss at operative site.

Mobility, impaired physical may be related to decreased strength, pain, musculoskeletal changes possibly evidenced by impaired coordination, and reluctance to attempt movement.

---

*Note: A potential diagnosis is not evidenced by signs and symptoms as the problem has not occurred and nursing interventions are directed at prevention.

Pain may be related to tissue trauma, local edema, surgical incision possibly evidenced by complaints of pain, narrowed focus, guarded movement, and autonomic responses (diaphoresis, changes in vital signs).

ARTHROSCOPY **MS**

Knowledge deficit [learning need] may be related to unfamiliarity with procedure/outcomes and self-care needs possibly evidenced by questions and requests for information.

ASTHMA **MS**

Airway clearance, ineffective may be related to increased pulmonary secretions and bronchospasm possibly evidenced by wheezing, tachypnea, and ineffective cough.

Gas exchange, impaired may be related to altered delivery of inspired oxygen possibly evidenced by restlessness, irritability, cyanosis, and changes in ABGs.

Anxiety (specify level) may be related to perceived threat of death possibly evidenced by apprehension, fearful expression, and extraneous movements.

PED

Activity intolerance may be related to imbalance between oxygen supply and demand possibly evidenced by fatigue and exertional dyspnea.

ATHLETE'S FOOT **CH**

Pain may be related to disruption of skin surface possibly evidenced by complaints of painful itching and restlessness.

*Infection, potential for spread** may be related to multiple breaks in skin exposure to moist/warm environment.

---

*See footnote on following page.

AUTISTIC DISORDER PSY/PED

Social interaction, impaired may be related to organic brain dysfunction, disturbance in self-concept, lack of bonding and development of trust, inadequate sensory stimulation or abnormal response to sensory input possibly evidenced by lack of responsiveness to others, lack of eye contact or facial responsiveness, treating persons as objects, lack of awareness of feelings in others, and indifference/aversion to comfort, affection, or physical contact.

Communication, impaired verbal may be related to organic brain dysfunction, psychologic barriers (inability to trust others, withdrawal into self, inadequate sensory stimulation, maternal deprivation) possibly evidenced by lack of interactive communication mode; does not use gestures or spoken language, absent or abnormal nonverbal communication; lack of eye contact or facial expression; peculiar patterns of speech (form, content, or speech production); and impaired ability to initiate or sustain conversation despite adequate speech.

*Violence, potential for, directed at self/others** may be related to organic brain dysfunction, inability to trust others, disturbance in self-concept, inadequate sensory stimulation or abnormal response to sensory input, maternal deprivation, and response to demands of therapy.

Family coping, ineffective, compromised/disabling may be related to chronic nature of disease and disability as well as parental supervision and lifestyle restrictions possibly evidenced by expression of despair, denial, depression, distortion of reality regarding the patient's condition, and protective behavior disproportionate to patient's abilities or need for autonomy.

---

*Note: A potential diagnosis is not evidenced by signs and symptoms as the problem has not occurred and nursing interventions are directed at prevention.

■ B

BATTERED CHILD SYNDROME PED/PSY

Self-esteem disturbance may be related to deprivation and negative feedback of family members possibly evidenced by lack of eye contact, withdrawal from social contacts, and discounting own needs.

Post-trauma response may be related to sustained/recurrent physical or emotional abuse possibly evidenced by acting-out behavior, development of phobias, poor impulse control, and emotional numbness.

Parenting, altered may be related to poor role model/identity, unrealistic expectations, presence of stressors, and lack of support possibly evidenced by verbalization of negative feelings, inappropriate caretaking behaviors, and evidence of physical/psychologic trauma to child.

Family coping, ineffective, compromised/disabled may be related to situational or developmental crisis and family disorganization possibly evidenced by verbalized concern about ability to deal with current situation and display of disproportionate (too little or too much) protective behaviors.

BIPOLAR DISORDER PSY

*Violence, potential for, directed at others/self** may be related to irritability and impulsive behavior and delusional thinking, angry response when ideas are refuted or wishes denied.

Nutrition, altered: Less than body requirements may be related to inadequate intake in relation to

---

*Note: A potential diagnosis is not evidenced by signs and symptoms as the problem has not occurred and nursing interventions are directed at prevention.

metabolic expenditures possibly evidenced by body weight 20 percent or more below ideal weight, observed inadequate intake, inattention to mealtimes, and distraction from task of eating.

*Poisoning, potential for (lithium toxicity)** related to narrow therapeutic range of drug, patient's ability to (or lack of) follow-through with medication regimen and monitoring, and denial of need for information/therapy.

Sleep pattern disturbance may be related to lack of recognition of fatigue/need to sleep, hyperactivity possibly evidenced by interrupted nighttime sleep, one or more nights without sleep, changes in behavior and performance, increasing irritability/restlessness, and dark circles under eyes.

Sensory-perceptual alteration, (specify/overload) may be related to decrease in sensory threshold, endogenous chemical alteration, psychologic stress, sleep deprivation possibly evidenced by increased distractibility and agitation, anxiety, disorientation, poor concentration, bizarre thinking, and motor incoordination.

Family processes, altered may be related to situational crises, illness, economics, change in roles, euphoric mood and grandiose ideas/actions, manipulative behavior and limit-testing, patient's refusal to accept responsibility for own actions possibly evidenced by statements of difficulty coping with situation, lack of adaptation to change or not dealing constructively with illness, ineffective family decision-making process, failure to send and to receive clear messages, and inappropriate boundary maintenance.

---

*Note: A potential diagnosis is not evidenced by signs and symptoms as the problem has not occurred and nursing interventions are directed at prevention.

BORDERLINE PERSONALITY DISORDER PSY

*Violence, potential for directed at self/others** may be related to use of projection as a major defense mechanism, pervasive problems with negative transference, and feelings of guilt/need to "punish" self.

Thought processes, altered may be related to psychologic conflicts and brief psychotic episodes, delusional thinking, cognitive distortions, increasing anxiety/fear, and poor reality base possibly evidenced by persecutory thoughts of "I am victim," perception of events as either grossly distorted or "did not happen at all," and interference with ability to think clearly and logically.

Self-esteem, disturbance/Role performance, altered may be related to lack of positive feedback, unmet dependency needs, retarded ego development, and fixation at an earlier level of development possibly evidenced by difficulty identifying self or defining self-boundaries, extreme mood changes, lack of tolerance of rejection or being alone, unhappiness with self, striking out at others, performance of ritualistic self-damaging acts, and belief that punishing self is necessary.

Anxiety (severe to panic) may be related to unconscious conflicts, perceived threat to self-concept, unmet needs possibly evidenced by transient psychotic symptoms, abuse of alcohol/other drugs, easy frustration and feelings of hurt, and performing self-mutilating acts.

Social isolation may be related to immature interests, unaccepted social behavior, inadequate personal resources, and inability to engage in satisfy-

---

*Note: A potential diagnosis is not evidenced by signs and symptoms as the problem has not occurred and nursing interventions are directed at prevention.

ing personal relationships possibly evidenced by difficulty meeting expectations of others; experiences feelings of difference from others, expresses interests inappropriate to developmental age, and shows behavior unaccepted by dominant cultural group.

BRAIN TUMORS MS

Pain may be related to pressure on brain tissues possibly evidenced by complaints of headache, facial mask of pain, narrowed focus, and autonomic responses (changes in vital signs).

Thought processes, altered may be related to altered circulation to and/or destruction of brain tissue possibly evidenced by memory loss, personality changes, and altered level of consciousness.

Sensory-perceptual alterations (specify) may be related to compression/displacement of brain tissue, disruption of neuronal conduction possibly evidenced by changes in visual acuity, alterations in sense of balance/gait disturbance, and paresthesia.

*Fluid volume deficit, potential** may be related to recurrent vomiting from irritation of vagal center in medulla, and decreased intake.

Self-care deficit (specify) may be related to sensory/neuromuscular impairment interfering with ability to perform tasks possibly evidenced by unkempt/disheveled appearance, body odor, and verbalization/observation of inability to perform activities of daily living.

BRONCHITIS CH

Airway clearance, ineffective may be related to excessive, thickened mucous secretions possibly

---

*Note: A potential diagnosis is not evidenced by signs and symptoms as the problem has not occurred and nursing interventions are directed at prevention.

evidenced by presence of rhonchi, tachypnea, and ineffective cough.

Activity intolerance may be related to imbalance between oxygen supply and demand possibly evidenced by complaints of fatigue, dypsnea, and abnormal vital sign response to activity.

Pain may be related to localized inflammation, persistent cough, aching associated with fever possibly evidenced by complaints, distraction behavior, and facial mask of pain.

BRONCHOPNEUMONIA MS

(Refer Also to Bronchitis)

Gas exchange, impaired may be related to inflammatory process and collection of secretions affecting exchange across alveolar membrane possibly evidenced by restlessness, dyspnea, cyanosis, and changes in mentation.

Hyperthermia may be related to infectious process and increased metabolic rate possibly evidenced by flushed warm skin, diaphoresis, tachypnea/tachycardia, and increased body temperature.

BURNS (DEPENDENT ON TYPE, DEGREE, AND SEVERITY OF THE INJURY) MS

Pain may be related to destruction of/trauma to tissue and nerves and edema formation possibly evidenced by verbal complaints of pain, narrowed focus, distraction behavior, and autonomic responses (changes in vital signs).

*Fluid volume deficit, potential** may be related to excessive losses through damaged capillaries and evaporation.

---

*Note: A potential diagnosis is not evidenced by signs and symptoms as the problem has not occurred and nursing interventions are directed at prevention.

*Infection, potential for** may be related to loss of protective dermal barrier, presence of necrotic tissue, altered immune response, and stress.

*Nutrition, altered: Less than body requirements, potential** may be related to presence of hypermetabolic state in response to burn injury/stress.

Skin integrity, impaired related to tissue trauma, disruption of skin surface with destruction of skin layers (partial/full-thickness burn) possibly evidenced by absence of viable tissue.

Post-trauma response may be related to life-threatening event possibly evidenced by re-experiencing the event, repetitive dreams/nightmares, psychic/emotional numbness, and sleep disturbance.

PED

Diversional activity deficit may be related to long-term hospitalization, frequent lengthy treatments, and physical limitations possibly evidenced by boredom, restlessness, withdrawal and requests for something to do.

Growth and development, altered may be related to effects of physical disability, separation from significant others, and environmental deficiencies possibly evidenced by loss of previously acquired skills and inability/reluctance to perform self-care.

BURSITIS **CH**

Pain may be related to inflammation of affected joint possibly evidenced by verbal complaints, guarding behavior, and narrowed focus.

Mobility, impaired physical may be related to inflammation and swelling of joint and pain possibly

---

*Note: A potential diagnosis is not evidenced by signs and symptoms as the problem has not occurred and nursing interventions are directed at prevention.

evidenced by diminished range of motion, reluctance to attempt movement, and imposed restrictions of movement by medical treatment.

■ C

CALCULI, URINARY — MS/CH

Pain may be related to tissue trauma and edema formation possibly evidenced by complaints of sudden, severe, colicky pain; and guarding and distraction behaviors.

*Urinary, retention, potential** may be related to obstruction of urinary flow.

*Infection, potential for** may be related to stasis of urine.

Knowledge deficit [learning need] may be related to lack of exposure/recall and information misinterpretation regarding condition, prognosis, and treatment needs possibly evidenced by requests for information, statements of concern, and recurrence/development of preventable complications.

CANCER — MS

(Refer Also to Chemotherapy)

Anxiety (specify level)/Fear may be related to change in health status, threat of death, threat to self-concept, and socioeconomic concerns possibly evidenced by feelings of inadequacy, helplessness, and fear; insomnia; and focus on self.

Grieving anticipatory may be related to potential loss (death) and perceived separation from significant others/lifestyle possibly evidenced by anger,

---

*Note: A potential diagnosis is not evidenced by signs and symptoms as the problem has not occurred and nursing interventions are directed at prevention.

sadness, withdrawal, and changes in eating/sleep patterns and activities.

Pain may be related to the disease process (compression of nerve tissue, infiltration of nerves or their vascular supply, obstruction of a nerve pathway, inflammation) possibly evidenced by complaints of pain, self-focusing/narrowed focus, alteration in muscle tone, facial mask of pain, distraction/guarding behaviors, autonomic responses, and restlessness.

PED

Family coping, ineffective compromised/disabling may be related to chronic nature of disease and disability, ongoing treatment needs, and parental supervision and lifestyle restrictions possibly evidenced by expression of denial/despair, depression, and protective behavior disproportionate to patient's abilities or need for autonomy.

*Family coping, potential for growth** may be related to the fact that the individual's needs are being sufficiently gratified and adaptive tasks effectively addressed, enabling goals of self-actualization to surface.

CH

Fatigue may be related to decreased metabolic energy production, increased energy requirements (hypermetabolic state), overwhelming psychologic/emotional demands, and altered body chemistry (side effects of medications, chemotherapy) possibly evidenced by unremitting/overwhelming lack of energy, inability to maintain usual routines, decreased performance, impaired ability to concen-

*Note: A potential diagnosis is not evidenced by signs and symptoms as the problem has not occurred and nursing interventions are directed at prevention.

trate, lethargy/listlessness, and disinterest in surroundings.

*Family process, altered, potential** may be related to situational transition and/or crises, long-term illness, changes in roles/economic status, and developmental transition (anticipated loss of a family member).

Home maintenance management, impaired may be related to debilitation, lack of resources, and/or inadequate support systems possibly evidenced by verbalization of problem, request for assistance, and lack of necessary equipment or aids.

CARDIAC SURGERY MS/PED

Anxiety (specify level)/Fear may be related to change in health status and threat to self-concept/death possibly evidenced by sympathetic stimulation, increased tension, and apprehension.

Knowledge deficit [learning need] may be related to lack of exposure/recall and misinterpretation of information possibly evidenced by verbalization of concern and request for information.

*Cardiac output, decreased, potential** may be related to decreased circulating fluid volume (preload), depressed myocardial contractility (pumping ability), changes in systemic vascular resistance (afterload), and alterations in electrical conduction.

Fluid volume deficit (2) [active loss] may be related to intraoperative bleeding with inadequate blood replacement; bleeding related to insufficient heparin reversal, fibrinolysis, or platelet destruction resulting from cardiopulmonary bypass pump; or volume depletion effects of intraoperative or postoperative diuretic therapy.

---

*Note: A potential diagnosis is not evidenced by signs and symptoms as the problem has not occurred and nursing interventions are directed at prevention.

*Gas exchange, impaired, potential** may be related to alveolar-capillary membrane changes (atelectasis), interstitial edema, inadequate function or premature discontinuation of chest tubes, and diminished oxygen-carrying capacity of the blood.

Pain may be related to tissue inflammation/edema formation (incisions), intraoperative nerve trauma, and myocardial ischemia possibly evidenced by complaints of incisional discomfort/pain, paresthesia/pain in hand, arm, shoulder; anxiety; restlessness; irritability; distraction behaviors and autonomic responses.

Skin/Tissue integrity, impaired related to mechanical trauma (surgical incisions, puncture wounds) and edema evidenced by disruption of skin surface.

CARPAL TUNNEL SYNDROME MS/CH

Pain may be related to pressure on median nerve possibly evidenced by complaints of pain, guarding behavior, and reluctance to use affected hand.

Mobility, impaired, physical may be related to neuromuscular impairment and pain possibly evidenced by decreased hand strength, limited range of motion, and reluctance to attempt movement.

Knowledge deficit [learning need] may be related to lack of exposure/recall and information misinterpretation regarding condition, prognosis, and treatment needs possibly evidenced by questions, statements of concern, request for information, and inaccurate follow-through of instructions/development of preventable complications.

---

*Note: A potential diagnosis is not evidenced by signs and symptoms as the problem has not occurred and nursing interventions are directed at prevention.

CAST (UPPER EXTREMITY) MS/CH

*Trauma, potential for additional injury** may be related to loss of skeletal integrity (fractures).

Pain may be related to movement of bone fragments, tissue trauma/edema, traction/immobility device, stress, and anxiety possibly evidenced by complaints of pain, distraction behaviors, self-focusing/narrowed focus, facial mask of pain, guarding/protective behavior, alteration in muscle tone, and autonomic responses.

Tissue perfusion, altered, peripheral may be related to reduction/interruption of blood flow: direct vascular injury, tissue trauma, excessive edema, thrombus formation, hypovolemia, edema formation possibly evidenced by cool, pale, or cyanotic fingers; delayed capillary refill; and complaints of numbness/tingling.

*Skin integrity, impaired potential** may be related to pressure of cast, moisture/debris under cast, and objects inserted under cast to relieve itching.

Self-care deficit (specify) may be related to impaired ability to perform self-care tasks possibly evidenced by statements of need for assistance and observed difficulty in performing activities of daily living.

CATARACT CH

Sensory-perceptual alteration, visual may be related to altered sensory reception/status of sense organs, and therapeutically restricted environment possibly evidenced by diminished acuity, visual distortions, and change in usual response to stimuli.

*Trauma, potential for** may be related to diminished visual acuity.

---

*Note: A potential diagnosis is not evidenced by signs and symptoms as the problem has not occurred and nursing interventions are directed at prevention.

Anxiety (specify level)/Fear may be related to alteration in visual acuity and threat of permanent loss of vision/independence possibly evidenced by feelings of uncertainty, apprehension, and expressed concerns.

Knowledge deficit [learning need] may be related to lack of information about ways of coping with altered abilities and therapy choices possibly evidenced by requests for information and statement of concern.

CAT SCRATCH DISEASE CH

Pain may be related to effects of circulating toxins (fever, headache, and lymphadenitis) possibly evidenced by complaints, guarding behavior, and autonomic response (changes in vital signs).

Hyperthermia may be related to inflammatory process possibly evidenced by increased body temperature, flushed warm skin, tachypnea, and tachycardia.

CEREBROVASCULAR ACCIDENT MS

Tissue perfusion, altered, cerebral may be related to interruption of blood flow (occlusive disorder, hemorrhage, cerebral vasospasm/edema) possibly evidenced by altered level of consciousness, memory loss, changes in motor/sensory responses, restlessness, language, intellectual and emotional deficits, and changes in vital signs.

Mobility, impaired physical may be related to neuromuscular impairment, decreased strength, and spasticity possibly evidenced by inability to purposefully move involved body parts, limited range of motion, and impaired coordination.

Swallowing, impaired may be related to muscle paralysis and perceptual impairment possibly evidenced by observed difficulty in swallowing, recurrent coughing, choking, and drooling.

Communication, impaired, verbal may be related

to motor and/or cognitive deficits possibly evidenced by garbled speech, inability to find and/or use correct words and identify objects and/or written/spoken words.

Sensory-perceptual alteration, (specify) may be related to altered sensory reception, transmission, integration (neurologic trauma or deficit), and psychologic stress (narrowed perceptual fields caused by anxiety), possibly evidenced by disorientation to time, place, and persons; changes in behavior pattern/usual response to stimuli; exaggerated emotional responses; poor concentration; bizarre thinking; reported/measured change in sensory acuity (hypoparesthesia); altered sense of taste/smell; inability to tell position of body parts (proprioception); inability to recognize/attach meaning to objects (visual agnosia); altered communication patterns; and motor incoordination.

*Neglect, unilateral, potential** may be related to sensory loss of part of visual field with perceptual loss of corresponding body segment.

Self-care deficit (specify) may be related to neuromuscular and/or cognitive impairment and depression possibly evidenced by stated/observed inability to perform activities of daily living, requests for assistance, disheveled appearance, and incontinence.

CH

Home maintenance management, impaired may be related to condition of individual family member, insufficient finances/family organization or planning, unfamiliarity with resources, and inadequate support systems possibly evidenced by members

*Note: A potential diagnosis is not evidenced by signs and symptoms as the problem has not occurred and nursing interventions are directed at prevention.

expressing difficulty in managing home in a comfortable manner/requesting assistance with home maintenance, disorderly surroundings, and overtaxed family members.

Health maintenance, altered may be related to lack of ability to make deliberate and thoughtful judgments, perceptual or cognitive impairment, and ineffective individual/family coping possibly evidenced by observed inability to take responsibility for meeting basic health practices/impairment of personal support system.

Body image/Role performance disturbance may be related to biophysical, psychosocial, and cognitive/perceptual changes possibly evidenced by actual change in structure and/or function, change in usual patterns of responsibility/physical capacity to resume role; and verbal/nonverbal response to actual or perceived change.

CESAREAN SECTION (ELECTIVE) OB

Knowledge deficit [learning need] may be related to incomplete/inadequate information regarding underlying procedure, pathophysiology, and care needs possibly evidenced by verbalization of concerns/misconceptions and inappropriate/exaggerated behavior.

Body image/Self-esteem disturbance may be related to required surgical intervention in an otherwise natural life event possibly evidenced by expressions of disappointment and negative feelings about body/self.

Anxiety (specify level) may be related to actual/perceived threat to mother/fetus, emotional threat to self-esteem, and unmet needs/expectations possibly evidenced by increased tension, restlessness, apprehension, uncertainty, fearfulness, feelings of inadequacy, sympathetic stimulation, trembling, and narrowed focus.

Pain may be related to presence of surgical incision and muscle contractions ("after pains") possibly evidenced by complaints, guarding/distraction behaviors and autonomic responses (changes in vital signs).

*Infection, potential for** may be related to interruption of skin barrier, invasive procedures, and delayed epithelialization at site of placental attachment.

CHEMOTHERAPY (CANCER) MS/CH

*Fluid volume deficit, potential** may be related to gastrointestinal losses and interference with adequate intake (stomatitis/anorexia).

Nutrition, altered: Less than body requirements may be related to inability to ingest adequate nutrients secondary to nausea, anorexia, and stomatitis possibly evidenced by weight loss, aversion to eating, reported altered taste sensation, and sore, inflamed buccal cavity.

Oral mucous membranes, altered may be related to effects of therapeutic regimen, dehydration, and malnutrition possibly evidenced by ulcerations, leukoplakia, decreased salivation, and complaints of pain.

Body image disturbance may be related to loss of hair and weight/body structure changes possibly evidenced by negative feelings, preoccupation with change, and change in social involvement.

CHOLECYSTECTOMY MS

Pain may be related to interruption in skin/tissue layers with mechanical closure (sutures/staples) and invasive procedures (including NG tube) possibly evidenced by complaints, guarding/distraction

---

*Note: A potential diagnosis is not evidenced by signs and symptoms as the problem has not occurred and nursing interventions are directed at prevention.

behaviors, and autonomic responses (changes in vital signs).

Oral mucous membranes, altered may be related to dehydration, mechanical trauma (NG tube) and mouth breathing possibly evidenced by dry mouth, coated tongue, complaints of discomfort, and decreased salivation.

Breathing patterns, ineffective may be related to decreased lung expansion secondary to pain and muscle weakness/ineffective cough possibly evidenced by fremitus, tachypnea, and decreased respiratory depth.

CHOLELITHIASIS CH

Pain may be related to inflammation and distention of tissues possibly evidenced by complaints, guarding/distraction behaviors, and autonomic responses (changes in vital signs).

Nutrition, altered: Less than body requirements may be related to inability to ingest/absorb adequate nutrients (food intolerance/pain, nausea/vomiting, anorexia) possibly evidenced by aversion to food/decreased intake and weight loss.

Knowledge deficit [learning need] may be related to lack of information about pathophysiology, therapy choices, and self-care needs possibly evidenced by verbalization of concerns, questions, and recurrence of condition.

CHRONIC OBSTRUCTIVE LUNG DISEASE MS

Airway clearance, ineffective may be related to increased production of tenacious secretions, retained secretions, decreased energy, and fatigue possibly evidenced by presence of rhonchi, tachypnea, dyspnea, pallor or cyanosis, and chest x-ray findings.

Gas exchange, impaired may be related to altered oxygen delivery (obstruction of airways by secretions/bronchospasm, air-trapping) and alveoli destruction possibly evidenced by dyspnea, confusion, restlessness, inability to move secretions, abnormal ABG values, changes in vital signs, and reduced tolerance for activity.

Activity intolerance may be related to imbalance between oxygen supply and demand possibly evidenced by verbal reports of fatigue, exertional dyspnea, and abnormal vital sign response.

Nutrition, altered: Less than body requirements may be related to inability to ingest adequate nutrients (dyspnea, fatigue, medication side effects, sputum production, anorexia, nausea/vomiting) possibly evidenced by weight loss, decreased muscle mass/subcutaneous fat, poor muscle tone, fatigue, reported altered taste sensation, aversion to eating, and lack of interest in food.

*Infection, potential for** may be related to decreased ciliary action, stasis of secretions, and debilitated state.

CIRRHOSIS — MS

Nutrition, altered: Less than body requirements may be related to inability to ingest/absorb nutrients (anorexia, nausea, indigestion, impaired storage of vitamins) possibly evidenced by aversion to eating, observed lack of intake, muscle wasting, and weight loss.

Fluid volume excess may be related to compromised regulatory mechanism (e.g., SIADH, decreased plasma proteins/malnutrition) and excess sodium/fluid intake possibly evidenced by edema/anasarca, weight gain, intake greater than output,

---

*Note: A potential diagnosis is not evidenced by signs and symptoms as the problem has not occurred and nursing interventions are directed at prevention.

changes in urine specific gravity, dyspnea, pleural effusion, and blood pressure changes.

*Skin integrity, impaired, potential** may be related to altered circulation/metabolic state, accumulation of bile salts in skin, poor skin turgor, skeletal prominence, and presence of edema/ascites.

*Thought processes, altered, potential** may be related to physiologic changes (increased serum ammonia level and inability of liver to detoxify certain enzymes/drugs).

Self-esteem/Body image, disturbance may be related to biophysical changes/altered physical appearance, uncertainty of prognosis, changes in role function, self-destructive behavior (alcohol-induced disease), and need for behavior/lifestyle changes possibly evidenced by verbalization of changes in lifestyle, fear of rejection or of reaction of others, negative feelings about body, and feelings of helplessness/hopelessness/powerlessness.

Knowledge deficit [learning need] may be related to lack of exposure/recall, information misinterpretation, and cognitive limitations possibly evidenced by questions, request for information, statement of misconception, and inaccurate follow-through of instruction/development of preventable complications.

COCAINE HYDROCHLORIDE POISONING PSY/MS

Thought processes, altered may be related to pharmacologic stimulation of the nervous system possibly evidenced by altered attention span, disorientation, and hallucinations.

Breathing pattern, ineffective may be related to

---

*Note: A potential diagnosis is not evidenced by signs and symptoms as the problem has not occurred and nursing interventions are directed at prevention.

pharmacologic effects on respiratory center of the brain possibly evidenced by tachypnea, altered depth of respiration, shortness of breath, and abnormal ABGs.

Coping, ineffective individual may be related to unwillingness to safely deal with actual/perceived stressors possibly evidenced by use of potentially harmful substance.

COCCIDIOIDOMYCOSIS (SAN JOAQUIN/VALLEY FEVER) CH

Pain may be related to inflammation possibly evidenced by complaints, distraction behaviors, and narrowed focus.

Fatigue may be related to decreased energy production; states of discomfort possibly evidenced by reports of overwhelming lack of energy, inability to maintain usual routine, emotional lability/irritability, impaired ability to concentrate, and decreased endurance/libido.

Knowledge deficit [learning need] may be related to lack of information about nature/course of disease and therapy needs possibly evidenced by statements of concern, and questions.

COLITIS, ULCERATIVE MS

(Refer Also to Crohn's disease)

Diarrhea may be related to inflammation, irritation or malabsorption of the bowel, toxins; segmental narrowing of the lumen possibly evidenced by increased bowel sounds/peristalsis, urgency, frequent/watery stools (acute phase), changes in stool color, and abdominal pain.

Pain may be related to inflammation of the intestines/hyperperistalsis and anal/rectal irritation possibly evidenced by complaints, guarding/distraction behaviors, and autonomic responses (changes in vital signs).

*Fluid volume deficit, potential** may be related to excessive gastrointestinal losses (diarrhea, capillary plasma loss), and altered intake.

Nutrition, altered: Less than body requirements may be related to altered intake/absorption of nutrients (medically restricted intake, fear that eating may cause diarrhea) and hypermetabolic state possibly evidenced by weight loss, decreased subcutaneous fat/muscle mass, poor muscle tone, hyperactive bowel sounds, steatorrhea, pale conjunctiva and mucous membranes, and aversion to eating.

Coping, ineffective, individual may be related to chronic nature and indefinite course of disease and inadequate handling of stressors possibly evidenced by altered ability to problem solve, verbalization of inability to cope, and presence of anxiety, depression, and exacerbation of symptoms.

CH

*Powerlessness, potential** may be related to unresolved dependency conflicts, feelings of insecurity/resentment, repression of anger and aggressive feelings, lacking a sense of control in stressful situations, sacrificing own wishes for others, and retreat from aggression or frustration.

COLOSTOMY MS

Skin integrity, impaired may be related to absence of sphincter at stoma and chemical irritation from caustic bowel contents possibly evidenced by erythema, excoriation of skin surrounding the stoma, and complaints of burning pain.

Diarrhea/Constipation (dependent on site) may

---

*Note: A potential diagnosis is not evidenced by signs and symptoms as the problem has not occurred and nursing interventions are directed at prevention.

be related to interruption/alteration of normal bowel function, changes in dietary/fluid intake, and effects of medication possibly evidenced by symptoms dependent on problem identified.

CH

Knowledge deficit [learning need] may be related to lack of exposure/recall, information misinterpretation regarding changes in physiologic function, and self-care/treatment needs possibly evidenced by questions, statement of concern, and inaccurate follow-through of instruction/development of preventable complications.

Social interaction, impaired may be related to fear of embarrassing situation secondary to altered bowel control with loss of contents, odor possibly evidenced by reduced participation and verbalized/observed discomfort in social situations.

*Sexual dysfunction, potential** may be related to altered body structure/function, radical resection/treatment procedures, vulnerability/psychologic concern about response of significant other(s), and disruption of sexual response pattern (e.g., erection difficulty).

Body image, disturbance may be related to biophysical changes (presence of stoma; loss of control of bowel elimination) and psychosocial factors (disease process/associated treatment regimen, i.e., cancer, colitis) possibly evidenced by verbalization of change in perception of self, negative feelings about body, fear of rejection/reaction of others, not touching/looking at stoma, and refusal to participate in care.

---

*Note: A potential diagnosis is not evidenced by signs and symptoms as the problem has not occurred and nursing interventions are directed at prevention.

CONCUSSION OF THE BRAIN MS

Pain may be related to trauma to/edema of cerebral tissue possibly evidenced by complaints of headache, guarding/distraction behaviors, and narrowed focus.

*Fluid volume deficit, potential** may be related to vomiting, decreased intake, and hypermetabolic state (fever).

CONGESTIVE HEART FAILURE MS

Cardiac output, decreased may be related to altered myocardial contractility/inotropic changes; alterations in rate, rhythm, and electrical conduction; and structural changes possibly evidenced by increased heart rate, changes in blood pressure, extra heart sounds, decreased urine output, diminished peripheral pulses, cool/ashen skin; diaphoresis, orthopnea, crackles, vascular distention, edema, and chest pain.

Activity intolerance may be related to imbalance between oxygen supply/demand, generalized weakness, and prolonged bedrest/immobility possibly evidenced by weakness, fatigue, changes in vital signs, presence of dysrhythmias, dyspnea, pallor, and diaphoresis.

Fluid volume, excess may be related to reduced glomerular filtration rate/increased ADH production, and sodium/water retention possibly evidenced by orthopnea, S_3 heart sound, oliguria, edema, jugular vein distention, positive hepatojugular reflex, weight gain, hypertension, respiratory distress, and abnormal breath sounds.

*Gas exchange, impaired, potential** may be re-

---

*Note: A potential diagnosis is not evidenced by signs and symptoms as the problem has not occurred and nursing interventions are directed at prevention.

lated to alveolar-capillary membrane changes (fluid collection/shifts into interstitial space/alveoli).

Knowledge deficit [learning need] may be related to lack of understanding/misconceptions about interrelatedness of cardiac function/disease/failure possibly evidenced by questions, statements of concern/misconceptions; and recurrent, preventable episodes of congestive heart failure.

CONN'S SYNDROME MS/CH

(Refer to Aldosteronism, Primary)

CONSTIPATION CH

Pain may be related to abdominal fullness/pressure, straining to defecate, and trauma to delicate tissues possibly evidenced by complaints, reluctance to defecate, and distraction behaviors.

Knowledge deficit [learning need] may be related to lack of understanding of dietary needs/bowel function possibly evidenced by development of problem and verbalization of concerns/questions.

CORONARY BYPASS MS

Cardiac output, decreased may be related to diminished circulating volume, alterations in electrical conduction, and increased systemic vascular resistance possibly evidenced by changes in hemodynamic readings, presence of ECG changes/dysrhythmias, and diminished peripheral pulses.

Fluid volume deficit, (2) [active loss] may be related to blood loss and intraoperative use of diuretics possibly evidenced by decreased right-sided filling pressures and blood pressure, concentrated urine with elevated specific gravity, dry mucous membranes, and decreased pulse volume/pressure.

Pain may be related to direct chest tissue/bone trauma, invasive tubes/lines, and donor site incision possibly evidenced by complaints, autonomic responses (changes in vital signs) and distraction behaviors.

Sensory-perceptual alterations, (specify) may be related to restricted environment, sleep deprivation, continuous environmental sounds/activities, and psychologic stress of procedure possibly evidenced by disorientation, alterations in behavior, exaggerated emotional responses, and visual/auditory distortions.

CROHN'S DISEASE MS/CH

(Refer Also to Colitis, Ulcerative)

Nutrition, altered: Less than body requirements may be related to postprandial pain and decreased transit time through bowel possibly evidenced by weight loss, aversion to eating, and observed lack of intake.

Diarrhea may be related to inflammation of small intestines, dietary intake possibly evidenced by hyperactive bowel sounds, cramping, and loose liquid stools of increased frequency.

Knowledge deficit [learning need] may be related to insufficient information/misinterpretation regarding pathophysiology of nutritional needs, and prevention of recurrence possibly evidenced by statements of concern, questions, and exacerbation of condition.

CROUP PED

Airway clearance, ineffective may be related to thick, tenacious mucous, and swelling/spasms of the epiglottis possibly evidenced by harsh/brassy cough, tachypnea, use of accessory muscles, and presence of rhonchi.

Fluid volume deficit, (2) [active loss] may be related to decreased ability/aversion to swallowing, presence of fever, and increased respiratory losses possibly evidenced by dry mucous membranes, poor skin turgor, and scanty/concentrated urine.

CROUP, MEMBRANEOUS PED

(Refer Also to Croup)

*Suffocation, potential for** may be related to inflammation of larynx with formation of false membrane.

Anxiety (specify level)/fear may be related to change in environment, perceived threat to self (difficulty breathing), and perception of anxiety of adults possibly evidenced by restlessness, facial tension, glancing about, and sympathetic stimulation.

CUSHING'S SYNDROME MS

Infection, potential for may be related to immunosuppressed inflammatory response, skin and capillary fragility, and negative nitrogen balance.

Nutrition, altered: Less than body requirements may be related to inability to utilize nutrients (disturbance of carbohydrate metabolism) possibly evidenced by decreased muscle mass and increased resistance to insulin.

Self-care deficit, (specify) may be related to muscle wasting, generalized weakness, fatigue, and demineralization of bones possibly evidenced by statements of/observed inability to complete or perform activities of daily living.

CH

Body image disturbance may be related to change in structure/appearance (effects of disease process, drug therapy) possibly evidenced by negative feelings about body, feelings of helplessness, and changes in social involvement.

Sexual dysfunction may be related to loss of li-

---

*Note: A potential diagnosis is not evidenced by signs and symptoms as the problem has not occurred and nursing interventions are directed at prevention.

bido, impotence, and cessation of menses possibly evidenced by verbalization of concerns and/or dissatisfaction and alteration in relationship with significant other.

*Trauma, potential for (fractures)** may be related to increased protein breakdown and negative protein balance.

CYSTIC FIBROSIS CH/PED

Airway clearance, ineffective may be related to excessive production of thick mucus and decreased ciliary action possibly evidenced by abnormal breath sounds, ineffective cough, cyanosis, and altered respiratory rate/depth.

*Infection, potential for** may be related to stasis of respiratory secretions and development of atelectasis.

Nutrition altered: Less than body requirements may be related to impaired digestive process and malabsorption of nutrients possibly evidenced by failure to gain weight, muscle wasting, and retarded physical growth.

Knowledge deficit [learning need] may be related to insufficient information concerning pathophysiology of condition, medical management, and available community resources possibly evidenced by statements of concern, questions, and misconceptions.

Family coping, ineffective, compromised may be related to chronic nature of disease and disability and parental supervision and lifestyle restrictions possibly evidenced by protective behavior disproportionate to patient's abilities or need for autonomy.

---

*Note: A potential diagnosis is not evidenced by signs and symptoms as the problem has not occurred and nursing interventions are directed at prevention.

CYSTITIS — CH

Pain may be related to inflammation and bladder spasms possibly evidenced by complaints, distraction behaviors, and narrowed focus.

Urinary elimination, altered may be related to inflammation/irritation of bladder possibly evidenced by frequency, nocturia, and dysuria.

Knowledge deficit [learning need] may be related to inadequate information regarding pathophysiology, treatment, and prevention of recurrence possibly evidenced by statements of concern and questions.

CYTOMEGALIC INCLUSION DISEASE — MS/CH

(Refer to Herpes Infections)

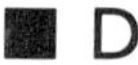

D

DEHISCENCE (ABDOMINAL) — MS

*Tissue integrity, impaired, potential** may be related to exposure of abdominal contents to external environment.

Skin integrity, impaired may be related to altered circulation, altered nutritional state (obesity/malnutrition), and physical stress on incision possibly evidenced by poor/delayed wound healing and disruption of skin surface/wound closure.

*Infection, potential for** may be related to inadequate primary defenses (separation of incision, traumatized intestines, environmental exposure).

Anxiety, acute may be related to perceived threat of death possibly evidenced by fearfulness, restless behaviors, and sympathetic stimulation.

---

*Note: A potential diagnosis is not evidenced by signs and symptoms as the problem has not occurred and nursing interventions are directed at prevention.

Knowledge deficit [learning need] may be related to lack of information/recall and misinterpretation of information possibly evidenced by development of preventable complication, requests for information, and statement of concern.

DEHYDRATION PED

Fluid volume deficit, (specify) may be related to etiology as defined by specific situation possibly evidenced by dry mucous membranes, poor skin turgor, decreased pulse volume/pressure, and thirst.

*Oral mucous membranes, altered, potential** may be related to dehydration and decreased salivation.

Knowledge deficit [learning need] may be related to lack of information, misinterpretation of fluid needs possibly evidenced by questions, statement of concern/misconceptions, and inadequate follow-through of instructions/development of preventable complications.

DELIRIUM TREMENS MS/PSY

Sensory-perceptual alterations, (specify) may be related to exogenous/endogenous chemical alterations, sleep deprivation, and psychologic stress possibly evidenced by disorientation, restlessness, irritability, exaggerated emotional responses, and visual and auditory distortions/hallucinations.

*Fluid volume deficit, potential** may be related to reduced intake, profuse diaphoresis, and agitation.

*Trauma, potential for** may be related to alterations in balance, reduced muscle coordination, and cognitive impairment.

Nutrition, altered: Less than body requirements,

---

*Note: A potential diagnosis is not evidenced by signs and symptoms as the problem has not occurred and nursing interventions are directed at prevention.

*potential** may be related to inability to absorb/utilize nutrients (depletion of liver glycogen stores, impaired gluconeogenesis), reduced intake, and debilitated state.

DEMENTIA, PRESENILE (ALZHEIMER'S) **MS**

Thought processes, altered may be related to cerebral neuronal degeneration possibly evidenced by memory deficit, decreased ability to grasp ideas/problem solve and make decisions, altered attention span, disorientation, delusions, and inappropriate social behavior/affect.

*Trauma, potential for** may be related to changes in muscle coordination/balance and cognitive difficulties.

Fear may be related to sensory impairment, physical deterioration, separation from support systems, and public disclosure of disabilities possibly evidenced by apprehension, irritability, defensiveness, suspiciousness, aggressive behavior, decreased self-assurance, and sympathetic stimulation.

Grieving, anticipatory may be related to early awareness of cognitive deficits and progressive permanent loss of abilities and self possibly evidenced by expressions of distress, anger, sorrow, and alterations in sleep and activity.

Self-care deficit, (specify) may be related to cognitive decline, physical limitations, frustration over loss of independence, and depression possibly evidenced by impaired ability to perform activities of daily living.

---

*Note: A potential diagnosis is not evidenced by signs and symptoms as the problem has not occurred and nursing interventions are directed at prevention.

CH

Family process, altered may be related to situational crisis; changing role responsibilities, relationships, and financial stability possibly evidenced by difficulty expressing feelings and problem solving and adapting or dealing with situation constructively.

Home maintenance management, impaired may be related to progressively impaired cognitive functioning, insufficient family organization/planning, unfamiliarity with resources, and inadequate support systems possibly evidenced by home surroundings appearing disorderly/unsafe, household members expressing difficulty and requesting help in maintaining home in safe/comfortable fashion, and overtaxed family members (e.g., exhausted/anxious).

Health maintenance, altered may be related to complete or partial lack of gross and/or fine motor skills, significant alteration in communication skills, and ineffective individual/family coping possibly evidenced by reported or observed inability to take responsibility for meeting basic health practices.

DEPRESSIVE DISORDERS, (MOOD DISORDERS) MAJOR DEPRESSION, DYSTHYMIA — PSY

*Violence, potential for, directed at self/others** may be related to depressed mood and feelings of worthlessness and hopelessness.

Coping, ineffective individual may be related to personal vulnerability, inadequate support systems, unrealistic perceptions, multiple life changes, inadequate coping method, unmet expectations, and ac-

*Note: A potential diagnosis is not evidenced by signs and symptoms as the problem has not occurred and nursing interventions are directed at prevention.

tual/perceived loss possibly evidenced by perception of events and stressors in a manner that precipitates depressive episode, perception of areas in life as unfulfilled or as losses, denial of loss, verbalization of inability to cope or ask for help, expression of guilt, crying/labile affect, and chronic anxiety/depression.

Sleep pattern, disturbance may be related to biochemical alterations (decreased serotonin), unresolved fears and anxieties, and inactivity possibly evidenced by difficulty in falling/remaining asleep, early morning awakening, complaints of not feeling rested, and dark circles under eyes.

Social isolation/Social interaction impaired may be related to alterations in mental status/thought processes, inadequate personal resources, decreased energy/inertia, difficulty engaging in satisfying personal relationships, feelings of worthlessness/low self-concept, inadequacy in/absence of significant purpose in life, and knowledge/skill deficit about social interactions possibly evidenced by decreased involvement with others, expressed feelings of difference from others, remaining in home/room/bed, refusing invitations/suggestions of social involvement, and dysfunctional interaction with peers, family and/or others.

Family processes, altered may be related to situational crises of illness of family member possibly evidenced by expressions of confusion, statements of difficulty coping with situation, family system not meeting needs of its members, difficulty accepting or receiving help appropriately, ineffective family decision-making process, and failure to send and to receive clear messages.

*Injury, potential for** may be related to electroconvulsive effects on the cardiovascular, respira-

---

*See footnote on following page.

tory, musculoskeletal, and nervous systems, and pharmacologic effects of anesthesia.

DIABETIC KETOACIDOSIS MS

Fluid volume deficit, (1) [regulatory failure] may be related to hyperosmolar urinary losses and inadequate intake possibly evidenced by dry mucous membranes, poor skin turgor, decreased pulse volume/pressure, and elevated temperature.

Nutrition, altered: Less than body requirements may be related to inadequate utilization of nutrients possibly evidenced by recent weight loss, reports of weakness, and imbalance between glucose/insulin levels.

*Breathing patterns, ineffective, potential** may be related to neuromuscular/musculoskeletal impairment and decreased energy levels.

*Infection, potential for** may be related to stasis of body fluids, invasive procedures, and alteration in circulation/perfusion.

DIABETES MELLITUS CH

Knowledge deficit [learning need] may be related to unfamiliarity with disease process/treatment and individual care needs possibly evidenced by requests for information, statements of concern/misconceptions, inadequate follow-through of instructions, and development of preventable complications.

Nutrition, altered: Less than body requirements may be related to inability to utilize nutrients (imbalance between intake and utilization of glucose) to meet metabolic needs possibly evidenced by

---

*Note: A potential diagnosis is not evidenced by signs and symptoms as the problem has not occurred and nursing interventions are directed at prevention.

change in weight, weakness, increased thirst/urination, and hyperglycemia.

*Adjustment, impaired, potential** may be related to all encompassing change in lifestyle and self-concept requiring lifelong adherence to therapeutic regimen and altered locus of control.

*Infection, potential for** may be related to decreased leukocytic phagocytosis, circulatory changes, and impaired healing.

DIALYSIS, PERITONEAL MS

Fluid volume excess may be related to excessive intake and/or fluid retention from dialysate drainage problems/inappropriate osmotic gradient of solution possibly evidenced by weight gain, edema, intake greater than output, and changes in blood pressure and respiratory pattern.

Pain may be related to factors related to procedure as well as presence of edema and required activity restrictions possibly evidenced by complaints (specify), distraction behaviors, and narrowed focus.

*Infection, potential for** may be related to compromised primary defenses, invasive procedures, and debilitated state.

*Breathing pattern, ineffective, potential** may be related to increased abdominal pressure with decreased lung expansion, pain/discomfort, and anxiety.

CH

Body image/role performance disturbance may be related to situational crisis and chronic illness with changes in usual roles possibly evidenced by

---

*Note: A potential diagnosis is not evidenced by signs and symptoms as the problem has not occurred and nursing interventions are directed at prevention.

verbalization of changes in lifestyle, focus on past function, negative feelings about body, feelings of helplessness/powerlessness, extension of body boundary to incorporate environmental objects (e.g., dialysis machine), change in social involvement, overdependence on others for care, not taking responsibility for self-care/lack of follow-through, and self-destructive behavior.

Grieving, anticipatory may be related to actual or perceived loss, chronic and/or fatal illness, and thwarted grieving response to a loss possibly evidenced by verbal expression of distress/unresolved issues, denial of loss; altered eating habits, sleep and dream patterns, activity levels, libido; crying, labile affect, feelings of sorrow, guilt, and anger.

Powerlessness may be related to illness-related regimen and health-care environment possibly evidenced by verbal expression of having no control, depression over physical deterioration, nonparticipation in care, anger, and passivity.

DIARRHEA PED

Pain may be related to abdominal cramping and irritation/excoriation of skin possibly evidenced by complaints (specify), facial grimacing, and autonomic responses.

*Fluid volume deficit, potential** may be related to excessive losses through GI tract.

Knowledge deficit [learning need] may be related to lack of information regarding causative/contributing factors and therapeutic needs possibly evidenced by statements of concern, questions, and development of preventable complications.

Skin integrity, impaired may be related to effects

---

*Note: A potential diagnosis is not evidenced by signs and symptoms as the problem has not occurred and nursing interventions are directed at prevention.

of excretions on delicate tissues possibly evidenced by complaints of discomfort and disruption of skin surface/destruction of skin layers.

DIGITALIS TOXICITY MS/CH

Cardiac output, decreased may be related to chemical alterations/interference with myocardial electrical activity possibly evidenced by changes in rate/rhythm/conduction (development/worsening of dysrhythmias).

*Fluid volume deficit, potential** may be related to excessive losses from vomiting/diarrhea and decreased intake.

Knowledge deficit [learning need] may be related to information misinterpretation and lack of recall possibly evidenced by inaccurate follow-through of instructions and development of preventable complications.

Thought processes, altered may be related to physiologic effects of toxicity/reduced cerebral perfusion and impaired judgment possibly evidenced by disorientation and confusion.

DILATION AND CURETTAGE

(Refer Also to Abortion, Spontaneous) **OB**

Knowledge deficit [learning need] may be related to unfamiliarity with surgical procedure, possible post-procedural complications, and therapeutic needs possibly evidenced by requests for information and statements of concern/misconceptions.

---

*Note: A potential diagnosis is not evidenced by signs and symptoms as the problem has not occurred and nursing interventions are directed at prevention.

DISRUPTIVE BEHAVIOR DISORDERS (CHILDHOOD/ADOLESCENCE) PSY/PED

Coping, ineffective, individual may be related to inadequate coping strategies, maturational crisis, multiple life changes, lack of control of impulsive actions, and personal vulnerability possibly evidenced by inappropriate use of defense mechanisms, inability to meet role expectations, poor self-esteem, failure to assume responsibility for own actions, and excessive smoking/drinking/drug use.

*Violence, potential for, directed at self/others** may be related to dysfunctional family system and loss of significant relationships.

Adjustment, impaired may be related to nonexistent or unsuccessful ability to be involved in problem solving or goal setting, losses connected with current and/or past occurrences in individual situation (e.g., loss of self-esteem, family member/friends), poor school performance, relocation, lack of movement toward independence, and difficulty limiting expectations of self possibly evidenced by ambivalence toward parent(s), anxiety, self-blame, anger, and feelings of rejection, assault to self-esteem, and altered locus of control.

CH

Family coping, ineffective, compromised/disabling may be related to excessive guilt, anger, or blaming among family members regarding child's behavior; parental inconsistencies; disagreements regarding discipline, limit-setting, and approaches; and exhaustion of parental resources (prolonged coping with disruptive child) possibly evidenced by

---

*Note: A potential diagnosis is not evidenced by signs and symptoms as the problem has not occurred and nursing interventions are directed at prevention.

unrealistic parental expectations, rejection or overprotection of child; and exaggerated expressions of anger, disappointment, or despair regarding child's behavior or ability to improve or change.

Social interaction, impaired may be related to retarded ego-development, low self-esteem, dysfunctional family system, and neurologic impairment possibly evidenced by difficulty waiting turn in games or group situations, doesn't seem to listen to what is being said, has difficulty playing quietly and maintaining attention to task or play activity, often shifting from one activity to another and interrupting or intruding on others.

DISSEMINATED INTRAVASCULAR COAGULATION MS

Anxiety (specify level)/fear may be related to sudden change in health status and threat of death possibly evidenced by sympathetic stimulation, restlessness, focus on self, and apprehension.

*Fluid volume deficit, potential** may be related to failure of regulatory mechanism (coagulation process) and active loss/hemorrhage.

Tissue perfusion, altered, (specify) may be related to alteration of arterial/venous flow by microemboli throughout circulatory system and hypovolemia possibly evidenced by changes in respiratory rate and depth, changes in mentation, decreased urinary output, and development of acral cyanosis/focal gangrene.

*Gas exchange, impaired, potential** may be related to reduced oxygen-carrying capacity, development of acidosis, fibrin deposition in microcirculation, and ischemic damage of lung parenchyma.

---

*Note: A potential diagnosis is not evidenced by signs and symptoms as the problem has not occurred and nursing interventions are directed at prevention.

Pain may be related to bleeding into joints/muscles, hematoma formation, and ischemic tissues with areas of acral cyanosis/focal gangrene possibly evidenced by complaints (specify), narrowed focus, alteration in muscle tone, distraction behaviors, restlessness, autonomic responses, and guarding behavior.

DISSOCIATIVE DISORDERS
(INCLUDING MULTIPLE PERSONALITY) **PSY**

Anxiety (severe/panic)/Fear may be related to maladaptation of ineffective coping continuing from early life, unconscious conflict(s), threat to self-concept, unmet needs, and phobic stimulus possibly evidenced by fragmentation of the personality, maladaptive response to stress, increased tension, feelings of inadequacy, and focus on self/projection.

*Violence, potential for, directed at self/others** may be related to depressed mood, conflicting personalities, panic states, and suicidal/homicidal behaviors.

Personal identity, disturbance in may be related to psychologic conflicts (dissociative state), childhood trauma/abuse, threat to physical integrity/self-concept, and underdeveloped ego possibly evidenced by confusion about sense of self, purpose or direction in life, memory loss, alteration in perception or experience of the self, loss of one's own sense of reality/the external world, poorly differentiated ego boundaries, and presence of more than one personality within the individual.

Family coping, ineffective, compromised may be related to multiple stressors repeated over period of time, prolonged progression of disorder that ex-

---

*Note: A potential diagnosis is not evidenced by signs and symptoms as the problem has not occurred and nursing interventions are directed at prevention.

hausts the supportive capacity of significant people, and temporary family disorganization and role changes possibly evidenced by significant other describing inadequate understanding or knowledge base that interferes with effective assistive or supportive behaviors, and marital conflict.

DIVERTICULITIS **CH**

Pain may be related to inflammation of intestinal mucosa, abdominal cramping, and presence of fever/chills possibly evidenced by complaints (specify), guarding/distraction behaviors, autonomic responses, and narrowed focus.

Diarrhea/Constipation (specify) may be related to altered structure/function and presence of inflammation possibly evidenced by signs and symptoms dependent on specific problem, e.g., increase/decrease in frequency of stools and change in consistency.

Knowledge deficit [learning need] may be related to lack of information about disease process, potential complications, and therapeutic needs possibly evidenced by statements of concern, request for information, and development of preventable complications.

Powerlessness, potential* may be related to chronic nature of disease process with recurrent episodes, in spite of cooperation with medical regimen.

DOWN SYNDROME

(Refer Also to Mental Retardation) **PED**

Growth and development, altered may be related to effects of physical/mental disability possibly evi-

---

*Note: A potential diagnosis is not evidenced by signs and symptoms as the problem has not occurred and nursing interventions are directed at prevention.

denced by altered physical growth, delay/inability in performing skills and self-care/self-control activities appropriate for age.

*Trauma, potential for** may be related to poor muscle tone/coordination, weakness, and cognitive difficulties.

Nutrition, altered: Less than body requirements may be related to poor muscle tone and protruding tongue possibly evidenced by weak and ineffective sucking and observed lack of adequate intake with weight loss/failure to gain.

*Family coping, potential for growth** may be related to situational/maturational crisis requiring incorporation of new skills into family dynamics.

*Grieving, dysfunctional, potential for** may be related to loss of "the perfect" child, chronic condition requiring long-term care, and unresolved feelings.

*Parenting, altered, potential** may be related to interference/delayed development of parenting, and attachment behaviors.

*Social isolation, potential** may be related to withdrawal from usual social interactions and activities, assumption of total child care, and becoming overindulgent/overprotective.

DYSMENORRHEA GYN

Pain may be related to exaggerated uterine contractability possibly evidenced by complaints (specify), guarding/distraction behaviors, narrowed focus, and autonomic responses (changes in vital signs).

*Mobility impaired, physical, potential** may be

---

*Note: A potential diagnosis is not evidenced by signs and symptoms as the problem has not occurred and nursing interventions are directed at prevention.

related to severity of pain and presence of secondary symptoms (nausea, vomiting, syncope, chills).

Coping ineffective, individual may be related to chronic, recurrent nature of problem, anticipatory anxiety, and inadequate coping methods possibly evidenced by muscular tension, headaches, general irritability, chronic depression, and verbalization of poor self-esteem.

DYSRHYTHMIA, CARDIAC MS

Cardiac output, decreased may be related to altered electrical conduction, and reduced myocardial contractility possibly evidenced by alterations in hemodynamic readings, ECG changes, fatigue, dyspnea, and syncope.

Anxiety (specify level) may be related to perceived threat of death possibly evidenced by increased tension, apprehension, and expressed concerns.

Pain may be related to ischemic cardiac muscle possibly evidenced by complaints of pain, narrowed focus, and autonomic responses (diaphoresis, changes in vital signs).

CH

Knowledge deficit [learning need] may be related to lack of information/understanding of medical condition/therapy needs and unfamiliarity with information resources possibly evidenced by questions, statement of misconception, failure to improve on previous regimen, and development of preventable complications.

*Activity intolerance, potential** may be related to

---

*Note: A potential diagnosis is not evidenced by signs and symptoms as the problem has not occurred and nursing interventions are directed at prevention.

imbalance between myocardial oxygen supply and demand, and cardiac depressant effects of certain drugs (beta-blockers, antidysrhythmics).

■ E

ECTOPIC PREGNANCY (TUBAL) OB

Pain may be related to distention/rupture of fallopian tube possibly evidenced by complaints (specify), guarding/distraction behaviors, facial mask of pain, and autonomic responses (diaphoresis, changes in vital signs).

*Fluid volume deficit, potential** may be related to hemorrhagic losses and decreased/restricted intake.

Anxiety (specify level) may be related to threat of death and possible loss of ability to conceive possibly evidenced by increased tension, apprehension, sympathetic stimulation, restlessness, and focus on self.

ECZEMA (DERMATITIS) CH

Pain may be related to cutaneous inflammation and irritation possibly evidenced by complaints (specify), irritability, and scratching.

*Infection, potential for** may be related to broken skin and tissue trauma.

Social isolation may be related to alterations in physical appearance possibly evidenced by expressed feelings of rejection and decreased interaction with peers.

---

*Note: A potential diagnosis is not evidenced by signs and symptoms as the problem has not occurred and nursing interventions are directed at prevention.

EDEMA, PULMONARY MS

Fluid volume, excess may be related to excessive fluid/sodium intake and decreased cardiac functioning possibly evidenced by dyspnea, presence of crackles (rales), pulmonary congestion on x-ray, restlessness, anxiety, and increased CVP.

Gas exchange, impaired may be related to altered blood flow and decreased alveolar-capillary exchange possibly evidenced by hypoxia, restlessness, and confusion.

Anxiety (specify level)/Fear may be related to perceived threat of death (inability to breathe) possibly evidenced by responses ranging from apprehension to panic state, restlessness, and focus on self.

EMPHYSEMA (COPD) MS

Airway clearance, ineffective may be related to increased tenacious secretions, decreased energy level, and muscle wasting possibly evidenced by abnormal breath sounds (rhonchi), ineffective cough, changes in rate/depth of respirations, and dyspnea.

Gas exchange, impaired may be related to alveolar capillary membrane changes possibly evidenced by hypercapnea, hypoxia, restlessness, and changes in mentation.

Activity intolerance may be related to imbalance between oxygen supply and demand possibly evidenced by reports of fatigue/weakness, exertional dyspnea, and abnormal vital sign response to activity.

---

*Note: A potential diagnosis is not evidenced by signs and symptoms as the problem has not occurred and nursing interventions are directed at prevention.

Nutrition, altered: Less than body requirements may be related to inability to ingest food because of shortness of breath, anorexia, and generalized weakness possibly evidenced by lack of interest in food, reported altered taste, and observed inadequate intake and weight loss.

CH

*Infection, potential for** may be related to inadequate primary defenses (stasis of body fluids, decrease of ciliary action), chronic disease process, and malnutrition.

Powerlessness may be related to illness-related regimen and health-care environment possibly evidenced by verbal expression of having no control, depression over physical deterioration, and nonparticipation in care, anger, and passivity.

ENCEPHALITIS **MS**

Pain may be related to inflammation/irritation of the brain and cerebral edema possibly evidenced by complaints of headache, distraction behaviors, restlessness, and autonomic response (changes in vital signs).

Hyperthermia may be related to increased metabolic rate, illness, and dehydration possibly evidenced by increased body temperature, flushed/warm skin, and increased pulse and respiratory rate.

*Fluid volume deficit, potential** may be related to increased losses through diaphoresis, hypermetabolic state, and decreased fluid intake.

*Trauma/Suffocation, potential for** may be re-

*Note: A potential diagnosis is not evidenced by signs and symptoms as the problem has not occurred and nursing interventions are directed at prevention.

lated to restlessness, clonic/tonic muscle activity, altered sensorium, and cognitive impairment.

ENDOCARDITIS — MS

Cardiac output, decreased may be related to inflammation of lining of heart and structural change in valve leaflets possibly evidenced by fatigue, changes in heart sounds, tachycardia, and variations in hemodynamic readings.

Anxiety (specify level) may be related to change in health status and threat of death possibly evidenced by apprehension, expressed concerns, and focus on self.

Pain may be related to generalized inflammatory process and embolic phenomena possibly evidenced by complaints, narrowed focus, distraction behaviors, and autonomic responses (changes in vital signs).

*Tissue perfusion, altered, (specify), potential** may be related to embolic interruption of arterial flow.

ENDOMETRIOSIS — GYN

Pain may be related to pressure of concealed bleeding/formation of adhesions possibly evidenced by complaints (specify), guarding/distraction behaviors, and narrowed focus.

Sexual dysfunction may be related to pain secondary to presence of adhesions possibly evidenced by verbalization of problem, and alteration in relationship with significant other(s).

Knowledge deficit [learning need] may be related to lack of information regarding pathophysiology of condition and therapy needs possibly evidenced by statements of concern and misconceptions.

---

*See footnote on following page.

ENTERITIS, REGIONAL (COLITIS/CROHN'S) (Refer to Colitis, Ulcerative and Crohn's) MS

EPIDIDYMITIS MS

Pain may be related to inflammation, edema formation, and tension on the spermatic cord possibly evidenced by complaints, guarding/distraction behaviors, and autonomic responses (changes in vital signs).

*Infection, potential for** spread may be related to inadequate primary defenses; insufficient knowledge to avoid spread of infection.

Knowledge deficit [learning need] may be related to lack of information about pathophysiology, outcome, and self-care needs possibly evidenced by statements of concerns, misconceptions, and questions.

EPILEPSY CH

*Trauma/Suffocation potential** may be related to tonic/clonic muscle activity and change in level of consciousness.

Fear may be related to unpredictable nature of condition and potential for harm possibly evidenced by decreased self-assurance, verbalization of concern, and withdrawal from social contacts/activities.

Body image disturbance may be related to perceived neurologic functional change/weakness possibly evidenced by negative feelings about "brain"/self, change in social involvement, feelings of helplessness, and preoccupation with perceived change or loss.

---

*Note: A potential diagnosis is not evidenced by signs and symptoms as the problem has not occurred and nursing interventions are directed at prevention.

■ F

FAILURE TO THRIVE PED

Nutrition, altered: Less than body requirements may be related to inability to ingest/digest/absorb nutrients (defects in organ function/metabolism, genetic factors), and physical deprivation/psychosocial factors possibly evidenced by weight loss/lack of appropriate weight gain, laboratory tests reflecting nutritional deficiency, poor muscle tone, and pale conjunctiva.

*Parenting altered, potential** may be related to lack of knowledge, inadequate bonding, unrealistic expectations for self/infant, and lack of appropriate response of child.

Knowledge deficit [learning need] may be related to lack of information about pathophysiology of condition, nutritional needs, growth expectations, and parenting skills possibly evidenced by verbalization of concerns, questions, misconceptions, and development of preventable complications.

FETAL ALCOHOL SYNDROME PED

*Injury, potential for CNS damage** may be related to external chemical factors (alcohol intake by mother), placental insufficiency, fetal drug withdrawal in utero/postpartum, and prematurity.

*Parenting, altered, potential** may be related to mental and/or physical illness, inability of mother to assume the overwhelming task of unselfish giving and nurturing, and presence of stressors (financial/legal problems).

---

*Note: A potential diagnosis is not evidenced by signs and symptoms as the problem has not occurred and nursing interventions are directed at prevention.

PSY

Coping, ineffective, individual (mother) may be related to personal vulnerability, low self-esteem, inadequate coping skills, and multiple stressors (repeated over period of time) possibly evidenced by inability to meet basic needs/role expectations/problem solve, and excessive use of drug(s).

Family coping, ineffective, Disabling may be related to lack of/insufficient support from others, mother's drug problem and treatment status, together with poor coping skills, lack of family stability/overinvolvement of parents with children and multigenerational addictive behaviors possibly evidenced by abandonment, rejection, neglectful relationships with family members, and decisions and actions by family that are detrimental.

FETAL DEMISE **OB**

Grieving, anticipatory may be related to loss of child and lack of resolution of previous grieving response possibly evidenced by expressions of distress, changes in eating habits, alterations in sleep patterns, crying, anger, and denial.

Spiritual distress may be related to challenged belief and value system (birth is supposed to be the beginning of life, not of death) and intense suffering possibly evidenced by questioning of religious beliefs, concern about purpose of life and death, and anger (may be directed at God for "letting this happen").

Role performance, altered may be related to situational crisis (perceived inadequacy in "normal" reproductive role), and unanticipated changes in parental roles possibly evidenced by expressed concern about parenting abilities, feelings of failure/guilt, and sense of inadequacy.

FRACTURES (CASTS) MS

Pain may be related to loss of skeletal integrity, soft-tissue trauma/swelling and muscle spasm possibly evidenced by complaints (specify), guarding/distraction behaviors, and autonomic responses (changes in vital signs).

*Tissue perfusion, altered, peripheral, potential** may be related to vascular injury, interruption of arterial/venous flow secondary to swelling and/or thrombus formation.

*Self-care deficit, (specify), potential** may be related to loss of function and restrictive treatment modality.

Knowledge deficit [learning need] may be related to lack of information about healing process, therapy requirements, and potential complications possibly evidenced by statements of concern, questions, and misconceptions.

CH

Mobility, impaired may be related to neuromuscular skeletal impairment, pain/discomfort, and restrictive therapies possibly evidenced by inability to purposefully move within the physical environment, imposed restrictions, reluctance to attempt movement, limited range of motion, and decreased muscle strength/control.

FROSTBITE

(Refer to Hypothermia) MS

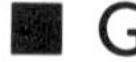

G

GALLSTONE

(Refer to Cholelithiasis) CH

---

*Note: A potential diagnosis is not evidenced by signs and symptoms as the problem has not occurred and nursing interventions are directed at prevention.

GANGRENE, DRY MS

Tissue perfusion, altered, peripheral may be related to interruption in arterial flow possibly evidenced by cool skin temperature, change in color (black), atrophy of affected part, and presence of pain.

Pain may be related to tissue hypoxia and necrotic process possibly evidenced by complaints (specify), guarding/distraction behaviors, narrowed focus, and autonomic responses (changes in vital signs).

GAS, LUNG IRRITANT MS/CH

Airway clearance, ineffective may be related to irritation/inflammation of airway possibly evidenced by marked cough, abnormal breath sounds (wheezes), dyspnea, and tachypnea.

Gas exchange, impaired, potential may be related to irritation/inflammation of alveolar membrane dependent on type of agent and length of exposure.

Anxiety (specific level) may be related to change in health status and threat of death possibly evidenced by increased tension, apprehension, and sympathetic stimulation.

GASTRITIS, ACUTE MS

Pain may be related to irritation/inflammation of gastric mucosa possibly evidenced by complaints (specify), guarding/distraction behaviors, and autonomic responses (changes in vital signs).

*Fluid volume deficit, potential** may be related to excessive losses through vomiting and diarrhea, reluctance to ingest fluids, and continued bleeding.

---

*Note: A potential diagnosis is not evidenced by signs and symptoms as the problem has not occurred and nursing interventions are directed at prevention.

GASTRITIS, CHRONIC **CH**

*Nutrition, altered: Less than body requirements, potential** may be related to inability to ingest adequate nutrients (prolonged nausea/vomiting, anorexia, epigastric pain).

Knowledge deficit [learning need] may be related to lack of information about pathophysiology, psychologic factors, therapy needs, and potential complications possibly evidenced by verbalizations of concerns, questions, misconceptions, and continuation of problem.

GASTROENTERITIS (GASTRITIS/ENTERITIS)

(Refer to Gastritis) **MS**

GENDER IDENTITY DISORDER **PSY**

Anxiety, severe may be related to unconscious/conscious conflicts about essential values/beliefs (ego-dystonic gender identification), threat to self-concept, and unmet needs possibly evidenced by increased tension, helplessness, hopelessness, feelings of inadequacy, uncertainty, insomnia, and focus on self.

Role performance altered/Personal identity disturbance may be related to crisis in development in which person has difficulty knowing to which sex s/he belongs; sense of discomfort and inappropriateness about anatomic sex possibly evidenced by confusion about sense of self, purpose or direction in life, sexual identification/preference, verbalization of desire to be/insistence that person is the opposite sex, change in self-perception of role, and conflict in roles.

---

*Note: A potential diagnosis is not evidenced by signs and symptoms as the problem has not occurred and nursing interventions are directed at prevention.

Sexuality patterns, altered may be related to ineffective or absent role models and conflict with sexual orientation and/or preferences possibly evidenced by verbalizations of discomfort with sexual orientation and/or role and lack of information about human sexuality.

*Family coping, ineffective compromised/disabling, potential** may be related to inadequate/incorrect information or understanding, temporary family disorganization and role changes, and patient providing little support in turn for primary person.

Family coping, potential for growth may be related to fact that individual's basic needs are sufficiently gratified and adaptive tasks effectively addressed to enable goals of self-actualization to surface possibly evidenced by family member(s) attempt(s) to describe growth/impact of crisis on own values, priorities, goals, or relationships; family member(s) is/are moving in direction of health-promotion and enriching lifestyle that supports patient's search for self; and choosing experiences that optimize wellness.

GLAUCOMA — MS/CH

Sensory-perceptual alteration, visual may be related to altered sensory reception and altered status of sense organ (increased intraocular pressure/atrophy of optic nerve head) possibly evidenced by progressive loss of visual field.

Anxiety (specify level) may be related to change in health status, presence of pain, possibility/reality of loss of vision, unmet needs, and negative self-talk possibly evidenced by apprehension, uncertainty,

*Note: A potential diagnosis is not evidenced by signs and symptoms as the problem has not occurred and nursing interventions are directed at prevention.

and expressed concern regarding changes in life events.

GLOMERULONEPHRITIS PED

Fluid volume, excess may be related to failure of regulatory mechanism (inflammation of glomerular membrane inhibiting filtration) possibly evidenced by weight gain, edema/anasarca, intake greater than output, and blood pressure changes.

Pain may be related to effects of circulating toxins and edema/distention of renal capsule possibly evidenced by complaints (specify), guarding/distraction behaviors, and autonomic responses (changes in vital signs).

Nutrition, altered: Less than body requirements may be related to anorexia and dietary restrictions possibly evidenced by aversion to eating, reported altered taste, weight loss, and decreased intake.

Diversional activity, deficit may be related to treatment modality, fatigue, and malaise possibly evidenced by statements of boredom, restlessness, and irritability.

GONORRHEA (STD) CH

*Infection potential for dissemination/bacteremia** may be related to presence of infectious process in highly vascular area and lack of recognition of disease process.

Pain may be related to irritation/inflammation of mucosa and effects of circulating toxins possibly evidenced by complaints (specify), guarding/distraction behaviors, and autonomic responses (changes in vital signs).

---

*Note: A potential diagnosis is not evidenced by signs and symptoms as the problem has not occurred and nursing interventions are directed at prevention.

Knowledge deficit [learning need] may be related to lack of information about disease cause/transmission, therapy, and self-care needs possibly evidenced by statements of concern, questions, misconceptions, and inaccurate follow-through of instructions/development of preventable complications.

GOUT CH

Pain may be related to inflammation of joint(s) possibly evidenced by complaints (specify), guarding/distraction behaviors, and autonomic responses (changes in vital signs).

Mobility, impaired physical may be related to joint pain/edema possibly evidenced by reluctance to attempt movement, limited range of motion, and therapeutic restriction of movement.

Knowledge deficit [learning need] may be related to lack of information about cause, treatment, and prevention of condition possibly evidenced by statements of concern, questions, misconceptions, and inaccurate follow-through of instructions.

GUILLAIN-BARRÉ SYNDROME MS

Mobility, impaired physical may be related to neuromuscular impairment possibly evidenced by decreased muscle strength/control, inability to purposefully move, and impaired coordination.

Anxiety (specify level) may be related to change in health status, threat to self-concept, and threat of death possibly evidenced by apprehension, feelings of depression, powerlessness, insomnia, and focus on self.

Sensory-perceptual alterations (specify) may be related to neurologic disease, sleep deprivation, therapeutically restricted environment, endogenous chemical alterations (electrolyte imbalance, hypoxia), and psychologic stress possibly evidenced by reported or observed change in usual response to stimuli, altered communication patterns, and measured change in sensory acuity and motor coordination.

*Breathing pattern ineffective, potential** may be related to neuromuscular impairment and decreased energy/lung expansion.

■ H

HAY FEVER — CH

Pain may be related to irritation/inflammation of upper airway mucous membranes and conjunctiva possibly evidenced by complaints (specify), irritability, and restlessness.

Knowledge deficit [learning need] may be related to lack of information regarding underlying cause and appropriate therapy and required lifestyle changes possibly evidenced by statements of concern, questions, and misconceptions.

HEATSTROKE — MS

Hyperthermia may be related to prolonged exposure to hot environment/vigorous activity with failure of regulating mechanism of the body possibly evidenced by high body temperature (above 105°F/40.6°C); flushed, hot skin; tachycardia; and seizures.

Cardiac output, decreased may be related to functional stress of hypermetabolic state, altered circulating volume/venous return, and direct myocardial damage secondary to hyperthermia possibly evidenced by decreased peripheral pulses, dysrhythmias/tachycardia, and changes in mentation.

---

*Note: A potential diagnosis is not evidenced by signs and symptoms as the problem has not occurred and nursing interventions are directed at prevention.

HEMODIALYSIS

MS

*Injury, potential for** may be related to multiple factors causing loss of vascular access (e.g., thrombosis, infection, disconnection/hemorrhage).

*Fluid volume deficit, potential** may be related to excessive fluid losses/shifts via ultrafiltration, hemorrhage from altered coagulation/disconnection of shunt, and fluid restrictions.

Body image disturbance may be related to change in function and dependence on mechanical support possibly evidenced by negative feelings about body, feelings of helplessness and powerlessness, change in social involvement, preoccupation with change, and possible extension of body boundary to incorporate environmental object.

*Nutrition, altered: Less than body requirements, potential** may be related to inadequate ingestion of nutrients (dietary restrictions, anorexia, nausea/vomiting, stomatitis).

CH

Powerlessness may be related to illness-related regimen and health-care environment possibly evidenced by verbal expression of having no control, depression over physical deterioration, nonparticipation in care, anger, and passivity.

Role performance, altered may be related to situational crisis and chronic illness with changes in usual roles possibly evidenced by verbalization of changes in lifestyle/usual responsibilities, change in physical capacity to resume role, focus on past function, overdependence on others for care, not taking responsibility for self-care/lack of follow-through, and self-destructive behavior.

---

*Note: A potential diagnosis is not evidenced by signs and symptoms as the problem has not occurred and nursing interventions are directed at prevention.

Coping, ineffective, individual may be related to situational crises/personal vulnerability, multiple life changes, inadequate support systems, and severe pain/overwhelming threat to self possibly evidenced by verbalization of inability to cope/asking for help, chronic worry, fatigue, insomnia, anxiety/depression, and inappropriate use of defense mechanisms.

Family coping, ineffective, compromised/disabling may be related to inadequate or incorrect information or understanding by a primary person, temporary family disorganization and role changes, patient providing little support in turn for the primary person, and prolonged disease/disability progression that exhausts the supportive capacity of significant persons possibly evidenced by expressions of concern or complaints about significant other's/family's response to patient's health problem, preoccupation of significant other(s) with own personal reactions, display of intolerance/rejection, and protective behavior disproportionate (too little or too much) to patient's abilities or need for autonomy.

HEMOPHILIA PED

*Fluid volume deficit, potential** may be related to hemorrhagic losses.

*Pain, chronic, potential** may be related to hemorrhage into joints.

*Mobility, impaired, physical, potential** may be related to joint hemorrhage, swelling, degenerative changes, and muscle atrophy.

Family coping, ineffective, compromised may be related to prolonged nature of condition that ex-

---

*Note: A potential diagnosis is not evidenced by signs and symptoms as the problem has not occurred and nursing interventions are directed at prevention.

hausts the supportive capacity of significant people possibly evidenced by protective behaviors disproportionate to patient's abilities/need for autonomy.

HEMOPTYSIS MS

Anxiety (specify level)/Fear **may be related to perceived threat of death possibly evidenced by apprehension, glancing about, facial tension, and statements of concern.**

Airway clearance, ineffective, potential* **may be related to collection of blood, mucus, and clot formation.**

Fluid volume deficit, potential* **may be related to excessive hemorrhagic losses.**

HEMORRHOIDECTOMY MS

Pain **may be related to edema/swelling and tissue trauma possibly evidenced by complaints, guarding/distraction behaviors, focus on self, and autonomic responses (changes in vital signs).**

Urinary retention, potential* **may be related to perineal trauma, edema/swelling, and pain.**

Knowledge deficit [learning need] **may be related to lack of information regarding therapeutic treatment and potential complications possibly evidenced by statements of concern and questions.**

HEMORRHOIDS OB/MS

Pain **may be related to inflammation and edema of prolapsed varices possibly evidenced by complaints (specify) and guarding/distraction behaviors.**

Constipation **may be related to pain on defecation**

---

*Note: A potential diagnosis is not evidenced by signs and symptoms as the problem has not occurred and nursing interventions are directed at prevention.

and reluctance to defecate possibly evidenced by frequency less than usual pattern and hard, formed stools.

HEMOTHORAX

(Refer Also to Pneumothorax) **MS**

*Trauma/Suffocation, potential for** may be related to concurrent disease/injury process, dependence on chest drainage system, and lack of safety education/precautions.

Anxiety (specify level) may be related to change in health status and threat of death possibly evidenced by increased tension, restlessness, expressed concern, sympathetic stimulation, and focus on self.

HEPATITIS (VIRAL) **MS**

Fatigue may be related to decreased metabolic energy production and altered body chemistry possibly evidenced by reports of lack of energy/inability to maintain usual routines, decreased performance, and increase in physical complaints.

Nutrition, altered: Less than body requirements may be related to inability to ingest adequate nutrients (nausea, vomiting, anorexia) possibly evidenced by aversion to eating/lack of interest in food, observed lack of intake, and weight loss.

Pain may be related to inflammation and swelling of the liver, urticarial eruptions, arthralgia, and pruritus possibly evidenced by complaints (specify), guarding/distraction behaviors, focus on self, and autonomic responses (changes in vital signs).

---

*Note: A potential diagnosis is not evidenced by signs and symptoms as the problem has not occurred and nursing interventions are directed at prevention.

CH

*Home maintenance management, impaired, potential** may be related to effects of disease process and inadequate support systems.

Knowledge deficit [learning need] may be related to lack of understanding about disease process/transmission, treatment needs, and future expectations possibly evidenced by questions, statement of concerns, inaccurate follow-through of instructions, and development of preventable complications.

HERNIATION OF NUCLEUS PULPOSUS MS

Pain may be related to nerve compression/irritation and muscle spasms possibly evidenced by complaints (specify), guarding/distraction behaviors, narrowed focus, and autonomic responses (changes in vital signs).

Mobility, impaired, physical may be related to pain and therapeutic restrictions/traction possibly evidenced by decreased muscle strength, limited range of motion, and reluctance to attempt movement.

Diversional activity, deficit may be related to lengthy hospitalization and therapy restrictions possibly evidenced by statements of boredom, disinterest, "nothing to do," and restlessness.

HERPES, HERPES SIMPLEX CH

Pain may be related to presence of localized inflammation and open lesions possibly evidenced by complaints (specify), distraction behaviors, and restlessness.

*Infection, potential for secondary infection** may

---

*Note: A potential diagnosis is not evidenced by signs and symptoms as the problem has not occurred and nursing interventions are directed at prevention.

be related to broken, traumatized tissue, and altered immune response.

*Sexuality, patterns altered, potential** may be related to fear of transmitting the disease.

HERPES NEONATAL

(Refer Also to Encephalitis) **PED**

*Nutrition, altered: Less that body requirements, potential** may be related to increased metabolic needs (infection) and inability to ingest nutrients (presence of vesicles in oral mucous membranes).

HERPES ZOSTER **CH**

Pain may be related to inflammation/local lesions along sensory nerve(s) possibly evidenced by complaints (specify), guarding/distraction behaviors, narrowed focus, and autonomic responses (changes in vital signs).

Knowledge deficit [learning need] may be related to lack of information about pathophysiology, therapeutic needs, and potential complications possibly evidenced by statements of concerns, questions, and misconceptions.

HIATAL HERNIA **CH**

Pain may be related to regurgitation of acidic gastric contents possibly evidenced by complaints (specify), facial grimacing, and focus on self.

Knowledge deficit [learning need] may be related to lack of information about pathophysiology and prevention of complications possibly evidenced by statements of concern, questions, and recurrence of condition.

---

*Note: A potential diagnosis is not evidenced by signs and symptoms as the problem has not occurred and nursing interventions are directed at prevention.

HIV-POSITIVE PATIENT CH

Knowledge deficit [learning need] may be related to lack of exposure, information misinterpretation, and unfamiliarity with accurate information resources possibly evidenced by statement of misconceptions/request for information, inappropriate or exaggerated behaviors (e.g., hysterical, hostile, agitated), and inaccurate follow-through of instructions.

HODGKIN'S DISEASE

(Refer Also to Cancer/Chemotherapy) MS

Knowledge deficit [learning need] may be related to lack of information about diagnosis, pathophysiology, treatment, and prognosis possibly evidenced by statements of concern, questions, and misconceptions.

Pain may be related to manifestations of inflammatory response (fever, chills, night sweats) and pruritus possibly evidenced by complaints (specify), distraction behaviors, and focus on self.

Anxiety (specify level)/Fear may be related to threat to self-concept and threat of death possibly evidenced by apprehension, insomnia, focus on self, and increased tension.

Nutrition, altered: Less than body requirements may be related to inability to ingest adequate nutrients (anorexia/dysphagia) possibly evidenced by weight loss, lack of interest in food, and observed decreased intake.

HYDROCEPHALUS PED

Tissue perfusion, altered, cerebral may be related to decreased arterial/venous blood flow (compression of brain tissue) possibly evidenced by changes in mentation, restlessness, irritability, complaints of headache, pupillary changes, and changes in vital signs.

Sensory-perceptual, alteration, visual may be related to pressure on sensory/motor nerves possibly evidenced by complaints of double vision, development of strabismus, nystagmus, pupillary changes, and optic atrophy.

Mobility, impaired, physical, potential may be related to neuromuscular impairment, decreased muscle strength, and impaired coordination.

CH

*Infection, potential for,** may be related to invasive procedure/presence of shunt.

Knowledge deficit [learning need] may be related to lack of understanding of condition, prognosis, and long-term therapy needs/medical follow-up possibly evidenced by questions, statement of concern, request for information, and inaccurate follow-through of instruction/development of preventable complications.

HYPERBILIRUBINEMIA **PED**

*Injury, potential for effects of treatment** may be related to adverse effects of phototherapy/exchange transfusions.

*Growth and development, altered, potential** may be related to effects of physical condition/collection of bilirubin in brain tissues (basal ganglia, brainstem nuclei).

Knowledge deficit [learning need] may be related to lack of exposure/recall and information misinterpretation possibly evidenced by questions, statement of concern, and inaccurate follow-through of instruction/development of preventable complications.

---

*Note: A potential diagnosis is not evidenced by signs and symptoms as the problem has not occurred and nursing interventions are directed at prevention.

HYPEREMESIS GRAVIDARUM OB

Fluid volume deficit, (2) [active loss] may be related to excessive gastric losses and reduced intake possibly evidenced by dry mucous membranes, decreased/concentrated urine, decreased pulse volume and pressure, thirst, and hemoconcentration.

Nutrition, altered: Less than body requirements may be related to inability to ingest/digest/absorb nutrients (prolonged vomiting) possibly evidenced by reported inadequate food intake, lack of interest in food/aversion to eating, and weight loss.

*Coping, ineffective, individual, potential** may be related to situational/maturational crisis (pregnancy, change in health status, projected role changes, concern about outcome).

HYPERTENSION MS

*Cardiac output, decreased, potential** may be related to increased afterload, (vasoconstriction), structural factors (increased systemic vascular resistance, myocardial ischemia, ventricular hypertrophy/rigidity).

Pain may be related to increased cerebral vascular pressure possibly evidenced by reports of throbbing pain located in suboccipital region, present on awakening and disappearing spontaneously after being up and about; reluctance to move head; avoidance of bright lights and noise; increased muscle tension; reports of dizziness; blurred vision; nausea; and vomiting.

CH

Knowledge deficit [learning need] may be related to lack of information/misinterpretation regarding

---

*Note: A potential diagnosis is not evidenced by signs and symptoms as the problem has not occurred and nursing interventions are directed at prevention.

pathophysiology, therapeutic regimen, lifestyle changes, and potential complications possibly evidenced by statements of concern/questions, inaccurate follow-through of instructions, and lack of control of condition.

Adjustment, impaired may be related to condition requiring change in lifestyle, altered locus of control, and absence of feelings of illness/denial possibly evidenced by verbalization of nonacceptance of health status change and lack of movement toward independence.

*Sexual dysfunction, potential** may be related to side effects of medication.

HYPERTHYROIDISM

(THYROTOXICOSIS) **CH**

Fatigue may be related to hypermetabolic imbalance with increased energy requirements, irritability of central nervous system, and altered body chemistry possibly evidenced by verbalization of overwhelming lack of energy to maintain usual routine, decreased performance, emotional lability/irritability, and impaired ability to concentrate.

Anxiety (specify level) may be related to increased stimulation of the central nervous system possibly evidenced by increased nervous tension, apprehension, irritability, and emotional lability.

*Nutrition, altered: Less than body requirements, potential** may be related to inability to ingest adequate nutrients for increased metabolic rate/constant activity or impaired absorption of nutrients (vomiting/diarrhea).

Tissue integrity, impaired may be related to pres-

---

*Note: A potential diagnosis is not evidenced by signs and symptoms as the problem has not occurred and nursing interventions are directed at prevention.

ence of periorbital edema and reduced ability to blink (protective mechanism) possibly evidenced by complaints of eye discomfort/dryness and development of corneal abrasion/ulceration.

HYPOGLYCEMIA CH

Thought processes, altered may be related to inadequate glucose for cellular brain function and effects of endogenous hormone activity possibly evidenced by irritability, changes in mentation, memory losses, altered attention span, and emotional lability.

*Nutrition, altered: Less than body requirements, potential** may be related to inadequate glucose metabolism and imbalance of glucose/insulin levels.

Knowledge deficit [learning need] may be related to lack of information/recall about pathophysiology of condition, and therapy/self-care needs possibly evidenced by development of hypoglycemia and statements of questions/misconceptions.

HYPOPARATHYROIDISM (ACUTE) MS

*Injury, potential for** may be related to neuromuscular excitability/tetany and formation of renal stones.

Pain may be related to recurrent muscle spasms and alteration in reflexes possibly evidenced by complaints (specify), distraction behaviors, and narrowed focus.

*Airway clearance ineffective, potential** may be related to spasm of the laryngeal muscles.

---

*Note: A potential diagnosis is not evidenced by signs and symptoms as the problem has not occurred and nursing interventions are directed at prevention.

HYPOTHERMIA (FROSTBITE) MS

Tissue integrity, impaired may be related to altered circulation and thermal injury possibly evidenced by damaged/destroyed tissue.

Pain may be related to diminished circulation with tissue ischemia/necrosis and edema formation possibly evidenced by complaints, guarding/distraction behaviors, narrowed focus, and autonomic responses (changes in vital signs).

*Infection, potential for** may be related to traumatized tissue/tissue destruction, and compromised immune response in affected area.

HYPOTHYROIDISM CH

Mobility, impaired, physical may be related to weakness, fatigue, muscle aches, altered reflexes, and mucin deposits in joints and interstitial spaces possibly evidenced by decreased muscle strength/control and impaired coordination.

Thought processes, altered may be related to actual physiologic changes with mucin deposits in interstitial spaces and decreased metabolic rate possibly evidenced by forgetfulness, impaired ability to conceptualize/reason, and personality changes.

Sensory-perceptual alterations, (specify) may be related to mucin deposits and nerve compression possibly evidenced by paresthesias of hands and feet or decreased hearing.

Constipation may be related to decreased peristalsis/physical activity possibly evidenced by frequency less than usual pattern; decreased bowel sounds; hard, dry stool; and development of fecal impaction.

---

*Note: A potential diagnosis is not evidenced by signs and symptoms as the problem has not occurred and nursing interventions are directed at prevention.

HYSTERECTOMY GYN/MS

Pain may be related to tissue trauma/abdominal incision possibly evidenced by complaints (specify), guarding/distraction behaviors, and autonomic responses (changes in vital signs).

*Urinary retention, potential** may be related to localized edema and nerve trauma with temporary bladder atony.

*Sexuality patterns, altered, potential** may be related to concerns regarding altered body function/structure.

■ I

ILEOCOLITIS

(Refer to Colitis) MS

ILEOSTOMY

(Refer to Colostomy) MS/CH

ILEUS MS

Pain may be related to distention/edema and ischemia of intestinal tissue possibly evidenced by complaints (specify), guarding/distraction behaviors, narrowed focus, and autonomic responses (changes in vital signs).

Diarrhea/Constipation may be related to presence of obstruction/changes in peristalsis possibly evidenced by changes in frequency and consistency or absence of stool, alterations in bowel sounds, presence of pain, and cramping.

*Fluid volume deficit, potential** may be related to

---

*Note: A potential diagnosis is not evidenced by signs and symptoms as the problem has not occurred and nursing interventions are directed at prevention.

increased intestinal losses (vomiting and diarrhea), and decreased intake.

IMPETIGO CH

Skin integrity impaired may be related to presence of infectious process and pruritus possibly evidenced by open/crusted lesions.

Pain may be related to inflammation and pruritus possibly evidenced by complaints (specify), distraction behaviors, and self-focusing.

*Infection, potential for secondary infection** may be related to broken skin, traumatized tissue, altered immune response, and virulence/contagious nature of causative organism.

*Infection, potential for transmission** to others may be related to virulent nature of causative organism.

INFLUENZA CH

Pain may be related to inflammation and effects of circulating toxins possibly evidenced by complaints (specify), distraction behaviors, and narrowed focus.

*Fluid volume, deficit, potential** may be related to excessive gastric losses, hypermetabolic state, and altered intake.

Hyperthermia may be related to effects of circulating toxins and dehydration, possibly evidenced by increased body temperature; warm, flushed skin; and tachycardia.

INSULIN SHOCK

(Refer to Hypoglycemia) CH

INTESTINAL OBSTRUCTION

(Refer to Ileus) MS

---

*Note: A potential diagnosis is not evidenced by signs and symptoms as the problem has not occurred and nursing interventions are directed at prevention.

■ K

KAWASAKI SYNDROME PED

Hyperthermia may be related to increased metabolic rate/illness and dehydration possibly evidenced by increased body temperature greater than normal range, flushed skin, increased respiratory rate, and tachycardia.

Pain may be related to inflammation and edema/swelling of tissues possibly evidenced by complaints (specify), restlessness, guarding behavior, and narrowed focus.

Skin integrity, impaired may be related to inflammatory process, altered circulation, and edema possibly evidenced by disruption of skin surface including macular rash and desquamation.

Oral mucous membranes, altered may be related to inflammatory process, dehydration, and mouth breathing possibly evidenced by pain, hyperemia, and fissures of lips.

*Cardiac output, decreased, potential** may be related to structural changes/inflammation of coronary arteries and alterations in rate/rhythm or conduction.

■ L

LABOR, INDUCED/AUGMENTED OB

*Injury, potential for maternal** may be related to deleterious effects of oxytocin administration, rapid labor, and delivery.

*Injury, potential for fetal** may be related to al-

*Note: A potential diagnosis is not evidenced by signs and symptoms as the problem has not occurred and nursing interventions are directed at prevention.

tered placental perfusion/cord relapse and precipitous delivery.

*Infection, potential for** may be related to rupture of amniotic membranes.

Knowledge deficit [learning need] may be related to lack of exposure/recall, information misinterpretation, and unfamiliarity with information resources possibly evidenced by questions, statement of concern/misconception, and inaccurate follow-through of instruction/development of preventable complications.

Pain may be related to rapid onset of strong, frequent contractions and level of anxiety possibly evidenced by complaints, distraction/guarding behaviors, and narrowed focus.

LABOR, STAGE I (ACTIVE PHASE) OB

Pain may be related to contraction-related hypoxia, dilation of the cervix, and pressure on adjacent structures combined with stimulation of both parasympathetic and sympathetic nerve endings possibly evidenced by complaints, distribution/guarding behaviors, and narrowed focus.

Urinary elimination, altered patterns may be related to retention of fluid in the prenatal period, increased glomerular filtration rate, decreased adrenal stimulation, dehydration, hemorrhage, severe intrapartal hypertension, pressure of the presenting part, and regional anesthesia possibly evidenced by increased/decreased output, decreased circulating blood volume, spasms of glomeruli and albuminuria, and reduced sensation.

*Coping, ineffective, individual/couple, potential**

---

*Note: A potential diagnosis is not evidenced by signs and symptoms as the problem has not occurred and nursing interventions are directed at prevention.

may be related to stressors accompanying labor, ineffective coping mechanisms, and pain.

*Self-esteem disturbance, potential** may be related to use of medications to relieve intense contractions and inability to carry out wish for an unmedicated childbirth.

LABOR, STAGE II (EXPULSION) OB

Pain may be related to strong uterine contractions, tissue stretching/dilation and compression of nerves by presenting part of the fetus, diaphoresis, and bladder distention possibly evidenced by complaints, facial grimacing, distraction/guarding behaviors, and narrowed focus.

Cardiac output, decreased may be related to repeated, prolonged Valsalva's maneuvers, effects of anesthesia/medications and dorsal recumbent position occluding the inferior vena cava and partially obstructing the aorta possibly evidenced by decreased venous return and changes in vital signs (blood pressure, pulse).

*Gas exchange, impaired, fetal, potential** may be related to head compression with vagal stimulation (causing bradycardia and hypoxia), cord compression, maternal position/prolonged labor affecting placental perfusion, and effects of maternal anesthesia.

*Skin, integrity, impaired, potential** may be related to untoward stretching/lacerations of delicate tissues (precipitous labor, hypertonic contractile pattern, adolescence, large fetus) and application of forceps.

Breathing pattern, ineffective may be related to anxiety, pain, decreased energy, and fatigue possi-

---

*Note: A potential diagnosis is not evidenced by signs and symptoms as the problem has not occurred and nursing interventions are directed at prevention.

bly evidenced by tachypnea, abnormal ABGs (maternal respiratory alkalosis), and changes in fetal heart rate/variability.

LAMINECTOMY (LUMBAR) MS

Tissue perfusion, altered (specify) may be related to diminished/interrupted blood flow; hypovolemia possibly evidenced by paresthesia, numbness, decreased range of motion, and muscle strength.

Pain may be related to incision, localized inflammation, and edema possibly evidenced by alteration in muscle tone, complaints (specify), and distraction/guarding behaviors.

Mobility, impaired physical may be related to imposed medical restrictions, decreased strength, and pain possibly evidenced by limited range of motion, decreased muscle strength, and reluctance to attempt movement.

Sensory-perceptual alteration, Kinesthetic, tactile may be related to inflammation/edema of compressed nerve or nerve root injury possibly evidenced by changes in sensation, movement, color, or temperature of lower extremities.

*Urinary retention potential** may be related to pain and swelling in operative area and reduced mobility.

LARYNGECTOMY

(RADICAL NECK SURGERY)

(Refer Also to Cancer, Chemotherapy) MS

Airway clearance, ineffective may be related to surgical trauma, partial/total removal of the glottis, which results in temporary or permanent neck breathing, edema formation, and copious and thick secretions possibly evidenced by dyspnea/difficulty

---

*Note: A potential diagnosis is not evidenced by signs and symptoms as the problem has not occurred and nursing interventions are directed at prevention.

breathing, changes in rate/depth of respiration, use of accessory respiratory muscles, weak/ineffective cough, abnormal breath sounds, and cyanosis.

Communication, impaired, verbal may be related to anatomic deficit (removal of vocal cords), physical barrier (tracheostomy tube), and required voice rest possibly evidenced by inability to speak, change in vocal characteristics, and impaired articulation.

Skin/Tissue integrity, impaired may be related to surgical removal of tissues/grafting, effects of radiation or chemotherapeutic agents, altered circulation/reduced blood supply, compromised nutritional status, edema formation, and pooling/continuous drainage of secretions possibly evidenced by disruption of skin surface and destruction of skin layers.

Oral mucous membranes, altered may be related to dehydration/absence of oral intake, poor/inadequate oral hygiene, pathologic condition (oral cancer), mechanical trauma (oral surgery), decreased saliva production secondary to radiation or surgical procedure, and nutritional deficits possibly evidenced by xerostomia (dry mouth), oral discomfort, thick/mucoid saliva, decreased saliva production, dry and crusted/coated tongue, inflamed lips, absent teeth/gums, and halitosis.

LARYNGITIS (CROUP)

(Refer to Croup) **CH/PED**

LEAD POISONING, ACUTE

(Refer Also to Lead Poisoning, Chronic) **PED**

*Trauma, potential for** may be related to loss of coordination, altered level of consciousness, and

---

*Note: A potential diagnosis is not evidenced by signs and symptoms as the problem has not occurred and nursing interventions are directed at prevention.

clonic or tonic muscle activity. (Continued exposure may lead to permanent neurologic damage.)

*Fluid volume deficit, (potential)** may be related to excessive vomiting, diarrhea, or decreased intake.

Knowledge deficit [learning need] may be related to lack of information about sources of lead and prevention of poisoning possibly evidenced by statements of concern, questions, and misconceptions.

LEAD POISONING, CHRONIC

(Refer Also to Lead Poisoning, Acute) **CH**

Nutrition, altered: Less than body requirements may be related to decreased intake (chemically induced changes in the gastrointestinal tract) possibly evidenced by anorexia, abdominal discomfort, reported metallic taste, and weight loss.

Thought processes, altered may be related to deposition of lead in central nervous system and brain tissue possibly evidenced by personality changes, learning disabilities, and impaired ability to conceptualize and reason.

Pain may be related to deposition of lead in soft tissues and bone possibly evidenced by complaints (specify), distraction behaviors, and focus on self.

LEUKEMIA, ACUTE

(Refer Also to Chemotherapy) **MS**

*Infection, potential for** may be related to inadequate secondary defenses (alterations in mature white blood cells, increased number of immature lymphocytes, immunosuppression and bone marrow suppression), invasive procedures, and malnutrition.

---

*Note: A potential diagnosis is not evidenced by signs and symptoms as the problem has not occurred and nursing interventions are directed at prevention.

Anxiety (specify level)/Fear may be related to change in health status, threat of death, and situational crisis possibly evidenced by apprehension, feelings of helplessness, and focus on self.

Activity intolerance may be related to imbalance between oxygen supply and demand possibly evidenced by generalized weakness, report of fatigue, exertional dyspnea, and abnormal vital sign response to activity.

Pain may be related to physical agents (infiltration of tissues/organs/central nervous system, expanding bone marrow) and chemical agents (antileukemic agents) possibly evidenced by complaints of abdominal discomfort, arthralgia, bone pain, headache, distraction behaviors, narrowed focus, and autonomic responses (changes in vital signs).

LONG-TERM CARE CH

Anxiety (specify level)/Fear may be related to change in health status, role functioning, interaction patterns, socioeconomic status, environment, unmet needs, recent life changes, and loss of friends/significant other(s) possibly evidenced by apprehension, restlessness, repetitive questioning, pacing, purposeless activity, and expressed concern regarding changes in life events.

Grieving, anticipatory may be related to perceived, actual, or potential loss of physiopsychosocial well-being, personal possessions, significant other(s) and cultural beliefs about aging possibly evidenced by denial of feelings, depression, sorrow, guilt, alterations in activity level, sleep patterns, eating habits, and libido.

*Poisoning, potential for drug toxicity** may be related to reduced metabolism, impaired circulation,

---

*Note: A potential diagnosis is not evidenced by signs and symptoms as the problem has not occurred and nursing interventions are directed at prevention.

precarious physiologic balance, presence of multiple diseases/organ involvement, and use of multiple prescribed/OTC drugs.

Thought processes, altered may be related to physiologic changes of aging, loss of cells and brain atrophy, decreased blood supply, altered sensory input, pain, effects of medications, and psychologic conflicts (disrupted life pattern) possibly evidenced by slower reaction times, gradual memory loss, altered attention span, disorientation, and inability to follow.

Sleep pattern, disturbance may be related to internal factors (illness, psychologic stress, inactivity), and external factors (environmental changes, facility routines) possibly evidenced by complaints of difficulty in falling asleep/not feeling well-rested, interrupted sleep, awakening earlier than desired, change in behavior/performance, increasing irritability, and listlessness.

*Skin integrity, impaired, potential** may be related to general debilitation, reduced mobility, changes in skin turgor and muscle mass associated with aging, sensory/motor deficits, altered circulation (edema, poor nutrition), excretions/secretions, and problems with self-care.

*Sexuality patterns, altered, potential** may be related to biopsychosocial alteration of sexuality, interference in psychologic/physical well-being, self-image, and lack of privacy/significant other(s).

LUPUS ERYTHEMATOSUS, SYSTEMIC CH

Pain may be related to widespread inflammatory process affecting connective tissues, blood vessels,

---

*Note: A potential diagnosis is not evidenced by signs and symptoms as the problem has not occurred and nursing interventions are directed at prevention.

serosal surfaces, and mucous membranes possibly evidenced by multiple complaints (specify), guarding/distraction behaviors, self-focusing, and autonomic responses (changes in vital signs).

Skin/Tissue integrity, impaired may be related to chronic inflammation, edema formation, and altered circulation possibly evidenced by presence of skin rash/lesions, ulcerations of mucous membranes, photosensitivity, and necrosis.

Fatigue may be related to increased energy requirements (chronic inflammation) and altered body chemistry (including effects of drug therapy) possibly evidenced by complaints of overwhelming lack of energy/inability to maintain usual routines, decreased performance, lethargy, and malaise.

Body image disturbance may be related to presence of chronic condition with rash, lesions, ulcers, purpura, mottled erythema of hands, alopecia, loss of strength, and altered body function possibly evidenced by hiding body parts, negative feelings about body, feelings of helplessness, and change in social involvement.

LYME DISEASE CH/MS

Pain may be related to systemic effects of toxins, presence of rash, urticaria, and joint swelling/inflammation possibly evidenced by complaints (specify), guarding behavior, autonomic responses, and narrowed focus.

Fatigue may be related to increased energy requirements, altered body chemistry, and states of discomfort possibly evidenced by complaints of overwhelming lack of energy/inability to maintain usual routines, decreased performance, lethargy, and malaise.

*Cardiac output, decreased, potential** may be related to alteration in rate/rhythm/conduction.

---

*See footnote on preceding page.

*Injury, potential for complications** may be related to external biologic factors (presence of spirochete) and failure to initiate prompt treatment.

■ M

MALLORY-WEISS SYNDROME MS

*Fluid volume deficit, potential** may be related to excessive vascular losses, presence of vomiting, and reduced intake.

Knowledge deficit [learning need] may be related to lack of information regarding causes, treatment, and prevention of condition possibly evidenced by statements of concern, questions, and recurrence of problem.

MASTECTOMY MS

Skin/Tissue integrity, impaired may be related to tension on suture line (removal of large amount of tissue, edema formation), altered circulation, and changes in skin elasticity/sensation, tissue destruction (radiation) possibly evidenced by disruption of skin surface, and destruction of skin layers/subcutaneous tissues.

Mobility impaired, physical may be related to pain, alteration in normal musculature/tissue integrity, and edema formation possibly evidenced by decreased muscle strength, limited range of motion, imposed medical restrictions, and reluctance to attempt movement.

Self-care deficit, bathing/dressing may be related to temporary loss/altered function of one or both arms possibly evidenced by statements of inability to perform/complete self-care tasks.

---

*Note: A potential diagnosis is not evidenced by signs and symptoms as the problem has not occurred and nursing interventions are directed at prevention.

Body image disturbance may be related to loss of body part denoting femininity possibly evidenced by not looking at/touching area, negative feelings about body, preoccupation with loss, and change in social involvement/relationship.

MASTITIS OB/GYN

Pain may be related to erythema and edema of breast tissues possibly evidenced by complaints (specify), guarding/distraction behaviors, self-focusing, and autonomic responses (changes in vital signs).

*Infection, potential for spread/abscess formation** may be related to traumatized tissues, stasis of body fluids, and insufficient knowledge to prevent complications.

Knowledge deficit [learning need] may be related to lack of information about pathophysiology, treatment, and prevention of complications possibly evidenced by statements of concern, questions, and misconceptions.

MASTOIDECTOMY MS

*Infection, potential for spread** may be related to pre-existing infection, surgical trauma, and stasis of body fluids in close proximity to brain.

Pain may be related to inflammation, tissue trauma, and edema formation possibly evidenced by complaints (specify), distraction behaviors, restlessness, self-focusing, and autonomic responses (changes in vital signs).

Sensory-perceptual alteration, auditory may be related to presence of packing, edema, and surgical disturbance of middle ear structures possibly evi-

---

*Note: A potential diagnosis is not evidenced by signs and symptoms as the problem has not occurred and nursing interventions are directed at prevention.

denced by reported/tested hearing loss in affected ear.

MEASLES CH/PED

Pain may be related to inflammation of mucous membranes, conjunctiva, and presence of extensive skin rash with pruritus possibly evidenced by complaints (specify), distraction behaviors, self-focusing, and autonomic responses (changes in vital signs).

Hyperthermia may be related to presence of viral toxins and inflammatory response possibly evidenced by increased body temperature, flushed/warm skin, and tachycardia.

*Infection, potential for, secondary** may be related to altered immune response and traumatized dermal tissues.

Knowledge deficit [learning need] may be related to lack of information about pathophysiology, transmission, and prevention of disease possibly evidenced by statements of concern, questions, misconceptions, and development of preventable complications.

MENINGITIS, ACUTE MS

Pain may be related to inflammation/irritation of the meninges with spasm of extensor muscles (neck, shoulders, and back) possibly evidenced by complaints (specify), guarding/distraction behaviors, narrowed focus, and autonomic responses (changes in vital signs).

Hyperthermia may be related to infectious process (increased metabolic rate) and dehydration

---

*Note: A potential diagnosis is not evidenced by signs and symptoms as the problem has not occurred and nursing interventions are directed at prevention.

possibly evidenced by increased body temperature, warm/flushed skin, and tachycardia.

*Trauma/Suffocation, potential for** may be related to alterations in level of consciousness, possible development of clonic/tonic muscle activity (seizures), and generalized weakness/prostration.

MENISCECTOMY MS

Mobility, impaired physical may be related to pain, joint instability, and imposed medical restrictions of movement possibly evidenced by decreased muscle strength/control, limited range of motion, and reluctance to attempt movement.

Knowledge deficit [learning need] may be related to lack of information about postoperative expectations, prevention of complications, and self-care needs possibly evidenced by statements of concern, questions, and misconceptions.

MENTAL RETARDATION

(Refer Also to Down Syndrome) **PED**

Communication, impaired, verbal may be related to developmental delay/impairment of cognitive and motor abilities possibly evidenced by impaired articulation, difficulty with phonation, and inability to modulate speech/find appropriate words (dependent on degree of retardation).

*Self-care deficit, (specify), potential** may be related to impaired cognitive ability and motor skills.

*Nutrition, altered, potential for more than body requirements** may be related to decreased metabolic rate coupled with impaired cognitive development and dysfunctional eating patterns.

Social interaction, impaired may be related to im-

---

*Note: A potential diagnosis is not evidenced by signs and symptoms as the problem has not occurred and nursing interventions are directed at prevention.

paired thought processes, communication barriers, and knowledge/skill deficit about ways to enhance mutuality possibly evidenced by dysfunctional interactions with peers, family and/or significant other(s), and verbalized/observed discomfort in social situations.

Family coping, ineffective, compromised may be related to chronic nature of disease and disability, parental supervision, and lifestyle restrictions possibly evidenced by protective behavior disproportionate to patient's abilities or need for autonomy.

CH

Home maintenance management, impaired may be related to impaired cognitive functioning, insufficient finances/family organization or planning, lack of knowledge, and inadequate support systems possibly evidenced by requests for assistance with home maintenance, expression of difficulty in maintaining home, disorderly surroundings, and overtaxed family members.

*Sexual dysfunction, potential** may be related to biopsychosocial alteration of sexuality, ineffectual/absent role models, misinformation/lack of knowledge, and lack of significant other(s).

MIGRAINE **CH**

Pain may be related to functional disturbance of cranial circulation possibly evidenced by complaints (specify), guarding/distraction behaviors, narrowed focus, and autonomic responses (changes in vital signs).

Mobility, impaired physical may be related to severe pain and intolerance to activity possibly evi-

---

*Note: A potential diagnosis is not evidenced by signs and symptoms as the problem has not occurred and nursing interventions are directed at prevention.

denced by reluctance to attempt movement, impaired coordination.

Knowledge deficit [learning need] may be related to lack of information regarding management of recurrent/temporarily debilitating condition possibly evidenced by statements of concern, questions, and misconceptions.

MITRAL STENOSIS MS

Activity intolerance may be related to imbalance between oxygen supply and demand possibly evidenced by reports of fatigue, weakness, exertional dyspnea, and tachycardia.

Gas exchange, impaired may be related to altered blood flow possibly evidenced by restlessness, hypoxia, and cyanosis (orthopnea/paroxysmal nocturnal dyspnea).

Knowledge deficit [learning need] may be related to lack of information regarding pathophysiology, therapeutic needs, and potential complications possibly evidenced by statements of concern, questions, inaccurate follow-through of instructions, and development of preventable complications.

MONONUCLEOSIS, INFECTIOUS CH

Fatigue may be related to decreased energy production, states of discomfort, and increased energy requirements (inflammatory process) possibly evidenced by reports of overwhelming lack of energy, inability to maintain usual routines, lethargy, and malaise.

Pain may be related to inflammation of lymphoid and organ tissues, irritation of oropharyngeal mucous membranes, and effects of circulating toxins possibly evidenced by complaints (specify), distraction behaviors, and self-focusing.

Hyperthermia may be related to inflammatory process possibly evidenced by increased body temperature, warm/flushed skin, and tachycardia.

Knowledge deficit [learning need] may be related to lack of information regarding disease transmission, self-care needs, medical therapy, and potential complications possibly evidenced by statements of concern, misconceptions, and inaccurate follow-through of instructions.

MOOD DISORDERS

(Refer to Depressive Disorders) **PSY**

MULTIPLE PERSONALITY

(Refer to Dissociative Disorders) **PSY**

MULTIPLE SCLEROSIS **CH**

Mobility, impaired physical may be related to neuromuscular and perceptual impairment and decreased strength and endurance possibly evidenced by impaired coordination, decreased muscle control and mass, and altered ability to move purposefully or perform routine tasks.

Sensory-perceptual alteration, visual, kinesthetic, tactile may be related to delayed/interrupted neuronal transmissions possibly evidenced by impaired vision, diplopia, disturbance of vibratory or position sense, paresthesias, numbness, and blunting of sensation.

Urinary elimination, altered patterns may be related to sensory-motor impairment possibly evidenced by frequency, nocturia, and incontinence.

Thought processes, altered may be related to physiologic changes, involvement of pathways of emotional control possibly evidenced by impaired judgment, emotional lability, and altered attention span.

Powerlessness/Hopelessness may be related to illness-related regimen, and lifestyle of helplessness possibly evidenced by verbal expressions of having no control or influence over the situation, depression over physical deterioration that occurs despite patient compliance with regimen, nonparticipation in care or decision making when opportunities are provided, passivity, decreased verbalization/affect, and lack of involvement in care/passively allowing care.

Home maintenance management, impaired may be related to effects of debilitating disease, impaired cognitive and/or emotional functioning, and inadequate support systems possibly evidenced by reported difficulty, observed disorderly surroundings, and poor hygienic conditions.

Family coping, compromised/disabling may be related to temporary family disorganization and role changes, situational crisis, patient providing little support in turn for significant other(s), prolonged disease/disability progression that exhausts the supportive capacity of significant other(s), feelings of guilt, anxiety, hostility, despair, and highly ambivalent family relationships possibly evidenced by patient expressing/confirming concern or complaint about significant other(s) response to patient's illness, significant other(s) preoccupied with own personal reactions, intolerance, abandonment, neglectful care of the patient, and distortion of reality regarding patient's illness.

MUMPS CH/PED

Pain may be related to presence of inflammation, circulating toxins, and enlargement of salivary glands possibly evidenced by complaints (specify), guarding/distraction behaviors, self-focusing, and autonomic responses (changes in vital signs).

Hyperthermia may be related to inflammatory process, increased metabolic rate, and dehydration possibly evidenced by increased body temperature, warm/flushed skin, and tachycardia.

*Fluid volume deficit, potential** may be related to

*See footnote on following page.

hypermetabolic state and painful swallowing with decreased intake.

MUSCULAR DYSTROPHY (DUCHENNE'S) PED

Mobility, impaired physical may be related to musculoskeletal impairment/weakness possibly evidenced by decreased muscle strength, control, and mass; limited range of motion; and impaired coordination.

Growth and development, altered may be related to effects of physical disability possibly evidenced by altered physical growth and altered ability to perform self-care/self-control activities appropriate to age.

*Nutrition, altered, potential for more than body requirements** may be related to sedentary lifestyle and dysfunctional eating patterns.

Family coping, compromised may be related to situational crisis/emotional conflicts around issues about hereditary nature of condition and prolonged disease/disability that exhausts supportive capacity of family members possibly evidenced by preoccupation with personal reactions regarding disability and displaying protective behavior disproportionate (too little/too much) to patient's abilities/need for autonomy.

MYASTHENIA GRAVIS MS

Breathing pattern/Airway clearance, ineffective may be related to neuromuscular weakness and decreased energy/fatigue possibly evidenced by dyspnea, changes in rate/depth of respiration, ineffective cough, and adventitious breath sounds.

---

*Note: A potential diagnosis is not evidenced by signs and symptoms as the problem has not occurred and nursing interventions are directed at prevention.

Communication, impaired verbal may be related to neuromuscular weakness, fatigue, and physical barrier (intubation) possibly evidenced by facial weakness, impaired articulation, hoarseness, and inability to speak.

Swallowing, impaired may be related to neuromuscular impairment of laryngeal/pharyngeal muscles and muscular fatigue possibly evidenced by reported/observed difficulty swallowing, coughing/choking, and evidence of aspiration.

Anxiety (specify level)/Fear may be related to situational crisis; threat to self-concept, change in health/socioeconomic status, role function, separation from support systems, lack of knowledge, and inability to communicate possibly evidenced by expressed concerns, increased tension, restlessness, apprehension, sympathetic stimulation, crying, focus on self, uncooperative behavior, withdrawal, anger, and noncommunication.

Sensory-perceptual alteration, visual may be related to neuromuscular impairment possibly evidenced by visual distortions (diplopia) and motor incoordination.

Knowledge deficit [learning need] may be related to inadequate information regarding drug therapy, potential for crisis (myasthenic or cholinergic) and self-care management possibly evidenced by statements of concern, questions, and misconceptions.

CH

Mobility, impaired, physical may be related to neuromuscular impairment possibly evidenced by reports of progressive fatigability with repetitive/prolonged muscle use, impaired coordination, and decreased muscle strength/control.

MYOCARDIAL INFARCTION

(Refer Also to Myocarditis) **MS**

Pain may be related to ischemia of myocardial tissue possibly evidenced by complaints (specify), guarding/distraction behaviors, facial mask of pain, self-focusing, and autonomic responses (diaphoresis, changes in vital signs).

Anxiety (specify level)/Fear may be related to threat of death, threat of change of health status, and role functioning and lifestyle possibly evidenced by increased tension, apprehension, expressed concerns, restlessness, and sympathetic stimulation.

Cardiac output, decreased may be related to changes in preload, systemic vascular resistance, electrical conduction, and muscle contractility/depressant effects of some drugs possibly evidenced by variations in hemodynamic readings, presence of ECG changes/dysrhythmias, cool/moist skin, and decreased peripheral pulses.

Activity intolerance may be related to imbalance between oxygen supply and demand and cardiac depressant effects of some drugs possibly evidenced by generalized weakness, exertional angina, abnormal heart rate/blood pressure responses, and development of dysrhythmias.

MYOCARDITIS MS

Activity intolerance may be related to imbalance with oxygen supply and demand and enforced bedrest possibly evidenced by reports of fatigue, exertional dyspnea, tachycardia/palpitations in response to activity, and ECG changes/dysrhythmias.

Knowledge deficit [learning need] may be related to lack of information regarding pathophysiology of condition and outcomes, medical therapy, and self-care needs/lifestyle changes possibly evidenced by statements of concern, misconceptions, inaccurate follow-through of instructions, and development of preventable complications.

MYRINGOTOMY

(Refer to Mastoidectomy) MS

MYXEDEMA (Hypothyroidism) CH

Body image disturbance may be related to change in structure/function (loss of hair/thickening of skin, mask-like facial expression, enlarged tongue, menstrual and reproductive disturbances) possibly evidenced by negative feelings about body, feelings of helplessness, and change in social involvement.

Nutrition, altered: More than body requirements may be related to decreased metabolic rate and activity level possibly evidenced by weight gain greater than ideal for height and frame.

*Cardiac output, decreased, potential** may be related to altered electrical conduction and myocardial contractility.

■ N

NEONATAL, NORMAL NEWBORN PED

*Gas exchange, impaired, potential** may be related to prenatal or intrapartal stressors, excess production of mucus, or cold stress.

*Body temperature, altered, potential** may be related to large body surface in relation to mass, limited amounts of insulating subcutaneous fat, nonrenewable sources of brown fat and few white fat stores, thin epidermis with close proximity of blood vessels to the skin, inability to shiver, and movement from a warm uterine environment to a much cooler environment.

Family processes, altered [bonding] may be related to developmental transition (gain of a family member) possibly evidenced by anxiety and excite-

---

*Note: A potential diagnosis is not evidenced by signs and symptoms as the problem has not occurred and nursing interventions are directed at prevention.

ment, expression of confusion/uncertainty, and difficulty accepting or receiving help appropriately.

*Nutrition, altered: Less than body requirements, potential** may be related to rapid metabolic rate, high caloric requirement, increased insensible water losses through pulmonary and cutaneous routes, and a potential for inadequate or depleted glucose stores.

*Infection, potential for** may be related to inadequate secondary defenses (deficiency of neutrophils and specific immunoglobulins), and inadequate primary defenses (traumatized tissues, decreased ciliary action).

NEONATAL, PREMATURE NEWBORN — PED

Gas exchange, impaired may be related to alveolar-capillary membrane changes (inadequate surfactant levels), altered blood flow (immaturity of pulmonary arteriole musculature), altered oxygen supply (immaturity of central nervous system and neuromuscular system, tracheobronchial obstruction), altered oxygen-carrying capacity of blood (anemia), and cold stress possibly evidenced by respiratory difficulties, inadequate oxygenation of tissues and acidemia.

Breathing pattern, ineffective may be related to decreased lung expansion/neuromuscular impairment (immaturity of the respiratory center, poor positioning, drug-related depression and metabolic imbalances), decreased energy/fatigue, inflammatory process, and tracheobronchial obstruction possibly evidenced by dyspnea, apneic spells, cyanosis,

---

*Note: A potential diagnosis is not evidenced by signs and symptoms as the problem has not occurred and nursing interventions are directed at prevention.

nasal flaring/use of accessory muscles, and abnormal ABGs.

*Thermoregulation, ineffective, potential** may be related to decreased ratio of body mass to surface area, decreased subcutaneous fat, inability to shiver or sweat, poor metabolic reserves, muted response to hypothermia, and frequent medical/nursing manipulations and interventions.

*Fluid volume deficit, potential** may be related to increased susceptibility to fluid losses (urine, feces, and insensible losses through lung and skin), thin skin and decreased insulating amounts of fat, immature kidney functioning, failure to conserve fluids during periods of dehydration, hypotension, and fluid shifts.

NEPHRECTOMY MS

Pain may be related to surgical tissue trauma and presence of incision with mechanical closure (suture) possibly evidenced by complaints (specify), guarding/distraction behaviors, self-focusing, and autonomic responses (changes in vital signs).

*Fluid volume, decreased, potential** may be related to excessive vascular losses and restricted intake.

Breathing pattern, ineffective may be related to incisional pain with decreased lung expansion possibly evidenced by tachypnea, fremitus, changes in respiratory depth/chest expansion, and changes in arterial blood gases.

Constipation may be related to reduced dietary intake, decreased mobility, gastrointestinal obstructions (paralytic ileus), and incisional pain with defecation possibly evidenced by decreased bowel

---

*Note: A potential diagnosis is not evidenced by signs and symptoms as the problem has not occurred and nursing interventions are directed at prevention.

sounds, reduced frequency/amount of stool, and hard/formed stool.

NEPHROTIC SYNDROME MS

Fluid volume, excess may be related to compromised regulatory mechanism with changes in hydrostatic/oncotic vascular pressure and increased activation of the renin-angiotension-aldosterone system possibly evidenced by edema/anasarca, effusions/ascites, weight gain, intake greater than output, and blood pressure changes.

Nutrition, altered: Less than body requirements may be related to excessive protein losses and inability to ingest adequate nutrients (anorexia) possibly evidenced by weight loss/muscle wasting (may be difficult to assess due to edema), lack of interest in food, and observed inadequate intake.

*Infection, potential for** may be related to chronic disease and steroidal suppression of inflammatory responses.

*Skin integrity, impaired, potential** may be related to presence of edema and activity restrictions.

NEURALGIA, TRIGEMINAL CH

Pain may be related to neuromuscular impairment with sudden violent muscle spasm possibly evidenced by complaints (specify), guarding/distraction behaviors, self-focusing, and autonomic responses (changes in vital signs).

Knowledge deficit [learning need] may be related to lack of information regarding control of recurrent episodes, medical therapies, and self-care needs possibly evidenced by statements of concern, questions, and exacerbation of condition.

---

*Note: A potential diagnosis is not evidenced by signs and symptoms as the problem has not occurred and nursing interventions are directed at prevention.

NEURITIS CH

Pain may be related to nerve damage usually associated with a degenerative process possibly evidenced by complaints (specify), guarding/distraction behaviors, self-focusing, and autonomic responses (changes in vital signs).

Knowledge deficit [learning need] may be related to lack of information regarding underlying causative factors, treatment, and prevention possibly evidenced by statements of concern, questions, and misconceptions.

■ O

OBESITY CH/PSY

Nutrition, altered: More than body requirements may be related to excessive intake in relation to metabolic needs possibly evidenced by weight 20 percent greater than ideal for height and frame, sedentary activity level, reported/observed dysfunctional eating patterns, and triceps skinfold greater than ideal for gender.

Body image disturbance may be related to mismatch between mental image and physical reality possibly evidenced by negative feelings about body, feelings of helplessness, and change in social involvement.

Activity intolerance may be related to imbalance between oxygen supply and demand and sedentary lifestyle possibly evidenced by fatigue or weakness, exertional discomfort, and abnormal heart rate in response to activity.

Coping, ineffective, individual may be related to personal vulnerability, unmet expectations, and inadequate coping method possibly evidenced by verbalization of difficulty dealing with anxiety and tension, overeating, and eating in response to stress.

OSTEOARTHRITIS
(ARTHRITIS, RHEUMATOID)

(Refer to Arthritis, Rheumatoid) **CH**

Note: Although this is a degenerative process versus inflammatory, nursing concerns are the same.

OSTEOMYELITIS **MS/CH**

Pain may be related to inflammation and tissue necrosis possibly evidenced by complaints (specify), guarding/distraction behaviors, self-focus, and autonomic responses (changes in vital signs).

Hyperthermia may be related to increased metabolic rate and infectious process possibly evidenced by increased body temperature and warm/flushed skin.

Tissue perfusion, altered, (bone) may be related to inflammatory reaction with thrombosis of vessels, destruction of tissue, edema, and abscess formation possibly evidenced by bone necrosis and continuation of infectious process and delayed healing.

Knowledge deficit [learning need] may be related to lack of information regarding pathophysiology of condition, long-term medical therapy, activity restrictions, and prevention of complications possibly evidenced by statements of concern, questions and misconceptions, and inaccurate follow-through of instructions.

OSTEOPOROSIS **CH**

Pain may be related to presence of fractures and vertebral compression on spinal nerves/muscles/

---

*Note: A potential diagnosis is not evidenced by signs and symptoms as the problem has not occurred and nursing interventions are directed at prevention.

ligaments possibly evidenced by complaints (specify), guarding/distraction behaviors, self-focus.

*Trauma, potential for** may be related to loss of bone integrity increasing risk of fracture with minimal or no stress.

Mobility, impaired physical may be related to pain and musculoskeletal impairment possibly evidenced by limited range of motion, reluctance to attempt movement, and imposed restrictions/limitations.

■ P

PALSY, CEREBRAL

(SPASTIC HEMIPLEGIA) **PED/CH**

Mobility, impaired physical may be related to muscular weakness/hypertonicity, increased deep tendon reflexes, tendency to contractures, and underdevelopment of affected limbs possibly evidenced by decreased muscle strength/control/mass, limited range of motion, and impaired coordination.

Family coping, compromised may be related to permanent nature of condition, situational crisis, emotional conflicts/temporary family disorganization, and incomplete information/understanding of patient's needs possibly evidenced by verbalized anxiety/guilt regarding patient's disability, inadequate understanding and knowledge base, and displaying protective behaviors disproportionate (too little/too much) to patient's abilities/need for autonomy.

Growth and development, altered may be related to effects of physical disability possibly evidenced by altered physical growth, delay or difficulty in performing skills (motor, social, expressive), and altered ability to perform self-care/self-control activities appropriate to age.

PANCREATITIS MS

Pain may be related to inflammation and edema of the pancreas with peritoneal irritation possibly evidenced by complaints (specify), guarding/distraction behaviors, self-focus, autonomic responses (changes in vital signs), and alteration in muscle tone.

*Fluid volume deficit, potential** may be related to excessive gastric losses (vomiting/nasogastric tube), hypermetabolic state, and hemorrhagic losses.

*Breathing pattern, ineffective, potential** may be related to inflammatory process/pain with decreased lung expansion.

Nutrition, altered: Less than body requirements may be related to medical restriction of intake as well as altered ability to digest nutrients possibly evidenced by weight loss and reduced muscle mass.

*Infection, potential for** may be related to inadequate primary defenses: stasis of body fluids, altered peristalsis, change in pH secretions, immunosuppression, nutritional deficiencies, tissue destruction, and chronic disease.

PARANOID DISORDERS PSY

*Violence, potential for, directed at self/others** may be related to perceived threats of danger and increased feelings of anxiety.

Anxiety, severe may be related to inability to trust (has not mastered tasks of trust versus mistrust) possibly evidenced by rigid delusional system (serves to provide relief from stress that justifies the delusion); frightened of other people and own hostility.

Powerlessness may be related to feelings of inad-

---

*Note: A potential diagnosis is not evidenced by signs and symptoms as the problem has not occurred and nursing interventions are directed at prevention.

equacy, interpersonal interaction, sense of severely impaired self-esteem, and belief that individual has no control over situation(s) possibly evidenced by use of paranoid delusions, use of aggressive behavior to compensate, and expressions of recognition of damage paranoia has caused self and others.

Thought processes, altered may be related to psychologic conflicts, increasing anxiety, and fear possibly evidenced by difficulties in the process and character of thought, interference with the ability to think clearly and logically, fragmentation and autistic thinking, and delusions.

Family coping, compromised may be related to temporary family disorganization/role changes, prolonged progression of condition that exhausts the supportive capacity of significant other(s) possibly evidenced by family system not meeting physical/emotional/spiritual needs of its members, inability to express or to accept wide range of feelings or feelings of members, and inappropriate boundary maintenance. Significant other(s) describes preoccupation with personal reactions.

PARAPLEGIA

(Refer Also to Quadriplegia) **MS/CH**

Mobility, impaired physical may be related to neuromuscular impairment (flaccid/spastic paralysis) possibly evidenced by loss of muscle control and coordination and inability to move purposefully.

Sensory-perceptual alterations, kinesthetic and tactile may be related to neurologic deficit with loss of sensory reception and transmission possibly evidenced by reported/measured change in sensory acuity and loss of usual response to stimuli.

Incontinence, reflex may be related to loss of nerve conduction above the level of the reflex arc possibly evidenced by lack of awareness of bladder filling/fullness, absence of urge to void, and uninhibited bladder contraction.

Body image disturbance/Role performance altered may be related to loss of body functions, change in physical ability to resume role, perceived loss of self/identity possibly evidenced by negative feelings about body/self, feelings of helplessness/powerlessness, delay in taking responsibility for self-care/participation in therapy, and change in social involvement.

Sexual dysfunction may be related to loss of sensation, altered function possibly evidenced by seeking of confirmation of desirability, verbalization of concern, and alteration in relationship with significant other.

PARATHYROIDECTOMY MS

Pain may be related to presence of surgical incision and effects of calcium imbalance (bone pain, tetany) possibly evidenced by complaints (specify), guarding/distraction behaviors, self-focus, and autonomic responses (changes in vital signs).

*Fluid volume excess, potential** may be related to preoperative renal involvement, stress-induced release of ADH, and changing calcium/electrolyte levels.

Airway clearance ineffective, potential* may be related to edema formation and laryngeal nerve damage.

Knowledge deficit [learning need] may be related to lack of information regarding postoperative care/complications and long-term needs possibly evidenced by statements of concern, questions, and misconceptions.

---

*Note: A potential diagnosis is not evidenced by signs and symptoms as the problem has not occurred and nursing interventions are directed at prevention.

PARKINSON'S DISEASE CH

Mobility, impaired physical may be related to neuromuscular impairment, (muscle weakness, tremors, bradykinesis) and musculoskeletal impairment (joint rigidity) possibly evidenced by decreased muscle strength/control, impaired coordination, and limited range of motion.

Swallowing, impaired may be related to neuromuscular impairment/muscle weakness possibly evidenced by reported/observed difficulty in swallowing, evidence of aspiration (choking, coughing, drooling).

Communication, impaired, verbal may be related to muscle weakness and incoordination possibly evidenced by impaired articulation, difficulty with phonation, and changes in rhythm and intonation.

PELVIC INFLAMMATORY DISEASE OB/GYN

*Infection, potential for spread** may be related to presence of infectious process in pelvic structures.

Pain may be related to inflammation, edema, and congestion of reproductive/pelvic tissues possibly evidenced by complaints (specify), guarding/distraction behaviors, self-focus, and autonomic responses (changes in vital signs).

Hyperthermia may be related to inflammatory process/hypermetabolic state possibly evidenced by increased body temperature, warm/flushed skin, and tachycardia.

Knowledge deficit [learning need] may be related to lack of information regarding cause/complications of condition, therapy needs, and transmission of disease to others possibly evidenced by statements of concern, questions, and misconceptions.

---

*Note: A potential diagnosis is not evidenced by signs and symptoms as the problem has not occurred and nursing interventions are directed at prevention.

PERIARTERITIS NODOSA

(Refer to Polyarteritis Nodosa) **MS/CH**

PERICARDITIS **MS**

Pain may be related to inflammation and presence of effusion possibly evidenced by complaints (specify), guarding/distraction behaviors, self-focus, and autonomic responses (changes in vital signs).

Activity intolerance may be related to imbalance between oxygen supply and demand possibly evidenced by complaints of weakness/fatigue, exertional dyspnea, abnormal heart rate or blood pressure response, and signs of congestive heart failure.

*Cardiac output, decreased, potential** may be related to accumulation of fluid (effusion) restricting cardiac filling/contractility.

Anxiety (specify level) may be related to change in health status and perceived threat of death possibly evidenced by increased tension, apprehension, restlessness, and expressed concerns.

PERIPHERAL VASCULAR DISEASE

(ATHEROSCLEROSIS) **CH**

Tissue perfusion, altered, peripheral may be related to reductions or interruptions of arterial/venous blood flow possibly evidenced by changes in skin temperature/color, lack of hair growth, blood pressure/pulse changes in extremity, presence of bruits, and complaints of claudication.

Activity intolerance may be related to imbalance between oxygen supply and demand possibly evidenced by reports of muscle fatigue/weakness and exertional discomfort (claudication).

*Tissue integrity impaired, potential** may be re-

---

*Note: A potential diagnosis is not evidenced by signs and symptoms as the problem has not occurred and nursing interventions are directed at prevention.

lated to altered circulation with decreased sensation and impaired healing.

PERITONITIS MS

*Infection, potential for spread/septicemia** may be related to inadequate primary defenses (broken skin, traumatized tissue, altered peristalsis), inadequate secondary defenses (immunosuppression), and invasive procedures.

Fluid volume deficit, (2) may be related to excessive gastric losses (vomiting, diarrhea, nasogastric tube), hypermetabolic state, and restricted intake possibly evidenced by dry mucous membranes, poor skin turgor, delayed capillary refill, weak peripheral pulses, diminished urinary output, dark/concentrated urine, hypotension, and tachycardia.

Pain may be related to inflammatory process and associated edema/distention of peritoneal tissues possibly evidenced by complaints (specify), guarding/distraction behaviors, self-focus, autonomic responses (changes in vital signs), and alterations in muscle tone.

Hyperthermia may be related to inflammatory process/hypermetabolic state, and dehydration possibly evidenced by increased body temperature, warm/flushed skin, and tachycardia.

PHEOCHROMOCYTOMA MS

Anxiety (specify level) may be related to excessive physiologic (hormonal) stimulation of the sympathetic nervous system possibly evidenced by apprehension, shakiness, restlessness, focus on self, fearfulness, diaphoresis, and sense of impending doom.

---

*Note: A potential diagnosis is not evidenced by signs and symptoms as the problem has not occurred and nursing interventions are directed at prevention.

Fluid volume deficit (1 and 2) may be related to excessive gastric losses (vomiting/diarrhea), hypermetabolic state, diaphoresis, and hyperosmolar diuresis possibly evidenced by hemoconcentration, dry mucous membranes, poor skin turgor, thirst, and weight loss.

Cardiac output, decreased/Tissue perfusion, altered (specify) may be related to altered preload/decreased blood volume, altered systemic vascular resistance, and increased sympathetic activity from excessive secretion of catecholamines possibly evidenced by cool/clammy skin, changes in blood pressure (hypertension/postural hypotension), visual disturbances, severe headache, and angina.

Knowledge deficit [learning need] may be related to lack of information regarding pathophysiology of condition, outcome, preoperative and postoperative care needs possibly evidenced by statements of concern, questions, and misconceptions.

PHLEBITIS

(Refer to Thrombophlebitis) **CH**

PHOBIA

(Refer Also to Anxiety) **PSY**

Fear may be related to learned irrational response to natural or innate origins (phobic stimulus) possibly evidenced by sympathetic stimulation and reactions ranging from apprehension to panic.

Social interaction, impaired may be related to intense fear of encountering feared object/activity or situation and anticipated loss of control possibly evidenced by reported change of style/pattern of interaction, discomfort in social situations, and avoidance of phobic stimulus.

---

*Note: A potential diagnosis is not evidenced by signs and symptoms as the problem has not occurred and nursing interventions are directed at prevention.

PLACENTA PREVIA — OB

*Fluid volume deficit, potential** may be related to excessive vascular losses.

Gas exchange, impaired, fetal may be related to altered blood flow, altered carrying capacity of blood (maternal anemia), and decreased surface area for gas exchange at site of placental attachment possibly evidenced by changes in fetal heart rate and activity and release of meconium.

Anxiety (specify level) may be related to situational crisis, threat to/change in health status (potential for hemorrhage/fetal death) possibly evidenced by increased tension, apprehension, uncertainty, sympathetic stimulation, restlessness, and narrowed focus.

*Diversional activity deficit, potential** may be related to imposed activity restrictions/bedrest.

PLEURISY — CH

Pain may be related to inflammation/irritation of the parietal pleura possibly evidenced by complaints (specify), guarding/distraction behaviors, self-focus, and autonomic responses (changes in vital signs).

Breathing pattern, ineffective may be related to pain on inspiration possibly evidenced by decreased respiratory depth, tachypnea, and dyspnea.

*Infection, potential for pneumonia** may be related to stasis of body fluids (pulmonary secretions), decreased lung expansion, and ineffective cough.

PNEUMONIA

(Refer to Bronchitis, Bronchopneumonia) **MS/CH**

---

*Note: A potential diagnosis is not evidenced by signs and symptoms as the problem has not occurred and nursing interventions are directed at prevention.

PNEUMOTHORAX MS

(Refer Also to Hemothorax)

Breathing pattern, ineffective may be related to decreased lung expansion possibly evidenced by dyspnea, tachypnea, altered chest excursion, respiratory depth changes, cough, cyanosis, and abnormal ABGs.

*Cardiac output, decreased, potential** may be related to compression/displacement of cardiac structures.

Pain may be related to irritation of nerve endings within pleural space by foreign object (chest tube) possibly evidenced by complaints (specify), guarding/distraction behaviors, self-focus, and autonomic responses (changes in vital signs).

POISONING (DRUG) MS/PED

Breathing pattern, ineffective may be related to depressant effect on central nervous system with cognitive impairment possibly evidenced by changes in respiratory depth, cyanosis, and abnormal ABGs.

*Poisoning, potential for** may be related to continued absorption and cumulative effects of ingested/injected drug(s).

*Violence, potential for, directed at self/others** may be related to suicidal behaviors and/or toxic reactions to drug(s).

PSY

Coping, ineffective, individual may be related to personal vulnerability, difficulty handling new situations, and previous ineffective/inadequate coping skills with substitution of drug(s) possibly evi-

---

*Note: A potential diagnosis is not evidenced by signs and symptoms as the problem has not occurred and nursing interventions are directed at prevention.

denced by denial, lack of acceptance that drug use is causing the present situation, altered social patterns/participation, impaired adaptive behavior and problem-solving skills, decreased ability to handle stress of illness/hospitalization, financial affairs in disarray, and employment difficulties.

POLYARTERITIS NODOSA MS/CH

Tissue perfusion, altered, (specify) may be related to reduction/interruption of blood flow possibly evidenced by organ tissue infarctions, changes in organ function, and development of organic psychosis.

Hyperthermia may be related to widespread inflammatory process possibly evidenced by increased body temperature and warm/flushed skin.

Pain may be related to inflammation, tissue ischemia, and necrosis of affected area possibly evidenced by complaints (specify), guarding/distraction behaviors, self-focus, and autonomic responses (changes in vital signs).

Grieving, anticipatory may be related to perceived loss of self possibly evidenced by expressions of sorrow and anger, altered sleep and/or eating patterns, changes in activity level, and libido.

POLYCYTHEMIA VERA CH

Activity intolerance may be related to imbalance between oxygen supply and demand possibly evidenced by reports of fatigue/weakness.

Tissue perfusion, altered, (specify) may be related to reduction/interruption of arterial/venous blood flow (insufficiency, thrombosis, or hemorrhage) possibly evidenced by pain in affected area, impaired mental ability, visual disturbances, and color changes of skin/mucous membranes.

POLYRADICULITIS

(Refer to Guillain-Barré) MS

POSTPARTAL PERIOD OB

*Family processes, altered, potential** may be related to developmental transition (gain of a family member) and transient period of disequilibrium.

*Fluid volume deficit, potential** may be related to excessive blood loss during delivery.

Pain may be related to incisional/perineal pain, afterpains, bladder fullness, and physical/psychologic exhaustion possibly evidenced by complaints, self-focusing, alteration in muscle tone, distraction behavior, and autonomic responses (changes in vital signs).

Urinary elimination, altered patterns may be related to physiologic return to nonpregnant state (decrease in circulating blood volume, continued elevation in renal plasma flow), mechanical trauma/tissue edema, and effects of medication/anesthesia possibly evidenced by frequency, dysuria, urgency, incontinence, or retention.

Constipation may be related to decreased muscle tone associated with diastasis recti, prenatal effects of progesterone, dehydration, excess analgesia or anesthesia, pain (hemorrhoids, episiotomy, or perineal tenderness), prelabor diarrhea, and lack of intake possibly evidenced by frequency less than usual pattern, hard-formed stool, straining at stool, decreased bowel sounds, and abdominal distention.

Sleep pattern disturbance may be related to discomfort, intense exhilaration/excitement, and anxiety possibly evidenced by verbal complaints of difficulty in falling asleep/not feeling well-rested, interrupted sleep, frequent yawning, and irritability.

---

*Note: A potential diagnosis is not evidenced by signs and symptoms as the problem has not occurred and nursing interventions are directed at prevention.

POSTOPERATIVE RECOVERY PERIOD MS/OB/GYN

Breathing pattern, ineffective may be related to neuromuscular, perceptual/cognitive impairment, decreased lung expansion/energy, and tracheobronchial obstruction possibly evidenced by changes in respiratory rate and depth, reduced vital capacity, apnea, cyanosis, and noisy respirations.

*Body temperature, altered, potential** may be related to exposure to cool environment, effect of medications/anesthetic agents, extremes of age/weight, and dehydration.

Sensory-perceptual alteration, (specify)/Thought processes, altered may be related to chemical alteration: use of pharmaceutical agents, hypoxia; therapeutically restricted environment; excessive sensory stimuli and physiologic stress possibly evidenced by changes in usual response to stimuli, motor incoordination, impaired ability to concentrate, reason, and make decisions; and disorientation to person, place, and time.

Pain may be related to disruption of skin, tissue, and muscle integrity, musculoskeletal/bone trauma, and presence of tubes and drains possibly evidenced by complaints, alteration in muscle tone, facial mask of pain, distraction/guarding behaviors, narrowed focus, and autonomic responses.

Skin/Tissue integrity, impaired may be related to mechanical interruption of skin/tissues, altered circulation, effects of medication, accumulation of drainage, and altered metabolic state possibly evidenced by disruption of skin surface/layers and tissues.

*Infection, potential for** may be related to broken

---

*Note: A potential diagnosis is not evidenced by signs and symptoms as the problem has not occurred and nursing interventions are directed at prevention.

skin, traumatized tissues, stasis of body fluids, presence of pathogens/contaminants, environmental exposure, and invasive procedures.

*Fluid volume, deficit, potential** may be related to restriction of oral intake, loss of fluid through abnormal routes (indwelling tubes, drains), normal routes (vomiting, loss of vascular integrity, changes in clotting ability), and extremes of age and weight.

POST-TRAUMATIC STRESS DISORDER PSY

Anxiety (severe to panic)/Fear may be related to current memory of past traumatic life event, threat to self-concept/death, change in environment, and negative self-talk possibly evidenced by increased tension/wariness, sense of helplessness, apprehension, fearfulness, uncertainty/confusion, restlessness, somatic complaints, sense of impending doom, and sympathetic stimulation with cardiovascular excitement/palpitations.

Powerlessness may be related to being overwhelmed by symptoms of anxiety and lifestyle of helplessness/poor coping skills possibly evidenced by verbal expression of lack of control over present situation/future outcome, reluctance to express true feelings, dependence on others, passivity and/or anger, and nonparticipation in care or decision making when opportunities are provided.

*Violence, potential for, directed at self/others** may be related to a startle reaction, an intrusive memory of an event causing a sudden acting-out of a feeling as if the event were occurring, use of alcohol/other drugs to ward off painful effects and pro-

---

*Note: A potential diagnosis is not evidenced by signs and symptoms as the problem has not occurred and nursing interventions are directed at prevention.

duce psychic numbing, breaking through of rage that has been walled off, response to intense anxiety or panic state, and loss of control.

Coping, ineffective, individual may be related to personal vulnerability, inadequate support system, unrealistic perceptions, unmet expectations, overwhelming threat to self, and multiple stressors repeated over period of time possibly evidenced by verbalization of inability to cope or difficulty asking for help, muscular tension/headaches, chronic worry, and emotional tension.

Grieving, dysfunctional may be related to actual/perceived object loss (loss of self as seen before the traumatic incident occurred as well as other losses incurred in/after the incident), loss of physiopsychosocial well-being, thwarted grieving response to a loss, and lack of resolution of previous grieving response possibly evidenced by verbal expression of distress at loss, anger, sadness, labile affect, alterations in eating habits/sleep and dream patterns/libido, reliving of past experiences, expression of guilt, and alterations in concentration.

Sleep pattern disturbance may be related to psychologic stress (anxiety, depression with recurring disruptive dreams) possibly evidenced by verbal complaints of difficulty in falling asleep/not feeling well-rested, insomnia, and reports of sleep disturbance (nightmares, dreams of personal death, disaster-related dreams, flashbacks, intrusive/trauma images, hypersomnia).

Family processes, altered may be related to situational crisis possibly evidenced by expressions of confusion about what to do and that they are having difficulty coping, family system not meeting physical/emotional/spiritual needs of its members, not adapting to change or dealing with traumatic experience constructively, and ineffective family decision-making process.

PREGNANCY-INDUCED HYPERTENSION — OB

Fluid volume deficit, (1) [regulatory failure] may be related to a shift of circulating volume from the vascular bed to interstitial space possibly evidenced by weight gain, edema formation, vasoconstriction, hemoconcentration, and altered serum sodium. (*Note:* Although signs of hypovolemia may be absent, the actual circulating volume is less than normal for pregnant state.)

Tissue perfusion, altered, renal may be related to decreased blood flow (vasoconstriction) and relative hypovolemia possibly evidenced by decreased urine output and abnormal laboratory values for renal function studies.

Gas exchange impaired/Nutrition, altered: Less than body needs, fetal may be related to vasospasm of spiral arteries and relative hypovolemia possibly evidenced by changes in fetal heart rate/activity, reduced weight gain, and premature delivery.

Knowledge deficit [learning need] may be related to lack of information regarding pathophysiology of condition, therapy, self-care/nutritional needs, and potential complications possibly evidenced by statements of concern, questions, and misconceptions.

THE PREGNANT ADOLESCENT

(Refer Also to Prenatal Period) — OB

Family processes, altered may be related to situational/developmental transition (economic, change in roles/gain of a family member) possibly evidenced by family expressing confusion about what to do, unable to meet physical/emotional/spiritual needs of the members, family inability to adapt to change or to deal with traumatic experience constructively, does not demonstrate respect for individuality and autonomy of its members, ineffective family decision-making process, and inappropriate boundary maintenance.

*Parenting, altered, potential** may be related to unmet social/emotional/maturational needs of parenting figures, unrealistic expectation of self/infant/partner, ineffective role model/social support, lack of role identity, and presence of stress (e.g., financial).

Social isolation may be related to restricted social sphere, stage of adolescence, and interference with accomplishing developmental tasks possibly evidenced by expressions of feelings of aloneness/rejection/difference from others, uncommunicative, withdrawn, no eye contact, seeking to be alone, unacceptable behavior, and absence of supportive significant other(s).

Body image/Self-esteem disturbance may be related to biophysical changes in body and change in life events possibly evidenced by fear of rejection/reaction of others, negative feelings about body, difficulty accepting positive reinforcement, and nonparticipation in prenatal care.

Knowledge deficit [learning need] may be related to lack of exposure, information misinterpretation, unfamiliarity with information resources about pregnancy, and sense of invulnerability/denial of reality possibly evidenced by questions, statement of concern/misconception, inaccurate follow-through of instruction, and development of preventable complications.

---

*Note: A potential diagnosis is not evidenced by signs and symptoms as the problem has not occurred and nursing interventions are directed at prevention.

PREMENSTRUAL (TENSION) SYNDROME GYN/CH

Pain may be related to vascular congestion/spasms possibly evidenced by complaints (specify), distraction behaviors, and self-focusing.

Fluid volume excess may be related to abnormal alterations of hormonal levels possibly evidenced by edema formation, weight gain, and changes in emotional status/irritability approximately one week before menstrual cycle.

Anxiety (specify level) may be related to cyclic changes in female hormones affecting other systems possibly evidenced by feelings of inability to cope/loss of control, depersonalization, increased tension, apprehension, jitteriness, somatic complaints, and impaired functioning.

Knowledge deficit [learning need] may be related to lack of information regarding pathophysiology of condition and self-care/treatment needs possibly evidenced by statements of concern, questions, misconceptions, and continuation of condition.

PRENATAL PERIOD (PREGNANCY) OB

*Nutrition, altered: Less than body requirements, potential** may be related to insufficient intake to meet increased metabolic demands (nausea/vomiting, inadequate financial/nutritional knowledge, increased thyroid activity associated with the growth of fetal and maternal tissues).

Pain may be related to hormonal influences causing minor discomforts possibly evidenced by complaints (nausea, breast changes, leg cramps, hemorrhoids, nasal stuffiness), alteration in muscle tone,

---

*Note: A potential diagnosis is not evidenced by signs and symptoms as the problem has not occurred and nursing interventions are directed at prevention.

restlessness, and autonomic responses (changes in vital signs).

*Injury, potential for, fetal** may be related to environmental/hereditary factors and problems of maternal well-being that directly affect the developing fetus.

*Cardiac output, decreased, potential** may be related to increased fluid volume/cardiac output and hormonal effects of progesterone and relaxin that place the patient at risk for hypertension and/or circulatory failure.

*Family coping, potential for growth** may be related to situational/maturational crisis with anticipated changes in family structure/roles.

*Constipation, potential for** may be related to changes in dietary/fluid intake, decreased peristalsis, and effects of medications (iron).

Sleep pattern disturbance may be related to internal factors (discomfort, anxiety, inactivity), external factors (demands of daily life) possibly evidenced by complaints of difficulty falling asleep/not feeling well-rested, interrupted sleep, irritability, lethargy, and frequent yawning.

*Role performance, altered, potential** may be related to difficulty adjusting to the overwhelming tasks associated with pregnancy/parenting, fear of injury to self/fetus, and weak ego.

Knowledge deficit [learning need] may be related to lack of information/recall of normal physiologic/psychologic changes, and misinterpretation possibly evidenced by questions, statement of concern, and inaccurate follow-through of instructions/development of preventable complications.

---

*Note: A potential diagnosis is not evidenced by signs and symptoms as the problem has not occurred and nursing interventions are directed at prevention.

PRETERM LABOR OB

Activity intolerance may be related to uteroplacental perfusion possibly evidenced by increase in uterine irritability and cervical dilatation.

*Poisoning, potential for** may be related to toxic side effects of treatments and medications used to stop labor.

*Injury, potential for fetal** may be related to premature birth.

Anxiety (specify level) may be related to perceived or actual threats to self/fetus and inadequate time to prepare for labor possibly evidenced by increased tension, restlessness, expressions of concern, and autonomic responses (changes in vital signs).

Knowledge deficit [learning need] may be related to lack of information about preterm labor, and misconceptions/misinterpretation possibly evidenced by questions, statement of concern, inaccurate follow-through of instruction, and development of preventable complications.

PROSTATE HYPERTROPHY, BENIGN MS/CH

Urinary elimination, altered may be related to obstruction of bladder outlet possibly evidenced by increasing urinary frequency, urgency, nocturia, incomplete bladder emptying, hesitancy, decrease in size/force of urinary stream, and post-void dribbling.

Pain may be related to mucosal irritation, bladder distention, renal colic, urinary infection, and radiation therapy possibly evidenced by complaints (bladder/rectal spasm), narrowed focus, altered

---

*Note: A potential diagnosis is not evidenced by signs and symptoms as the problem has not occurred and nursing interventions are directed at prevention.

muscle tone, grimacing, distraction behaviors, restlessness, and autonomic responses.

Sleep pattern disturbance may be related to urinary frequency and nocturia possibly evidenced by complaints of interrupted sleep/not feeling well-rested and irritability.

*Infection, potential for** may be related to urinary stasis.

Fear/Anxiety (specify level) may be related to change in health status (possibility of surgical procedure/malignancy); embarrassment/loss of dignity associated with genital exposure before, during, and after treatment; and concern about sexual ability possibly evidenced by increased tension, apprehension, worry, expressed concerns regarding perceived changes, and fear of unspecific consequences.

PROSTATECTOMY MS

Pain may be related to irritation of bladder mucosa and tissue trauma/edema possibly evidenced by complaints (specify), distraction behaviors, self-focus, and autonomic responses (changes in vital signs).

*Fluid volume deficit, potential** may be related to trauma to highly vascular area with excessive vascular losses.

Body image disturbance may be related to perceived threat of altered body/sexual function possibly evidenced by preoccupation with change/loss, negative feelings about body and statements of concern regarding functioning.

Urinary elimination, altered patterns may be related to mechanical trauma, mucosal irritation, and

---

*Note: A potential diagnosis is not evidenced by signs and symptoms as the problem has not occurred and nursing interventions are directed at prevention.

neuromuscular impairment possibly evidenced by dysuria, frequency, dribbling, and incontinence.

*Sexual dysfunction, potential** may be related to situational crisis (incontinence, leakage of urine after catheter removal, involvement of genital area) and threat to self-concept/change in health status.

PRURITUS CH

Pain may be related to cutaneous hyperesthesia and inflammation possibly evidenced by complaints (specify), distraction behaviors, and self-focus.

*Skin integrity, impaired, potential** may be related to mechanical trauma (scratching) and development of vesicles/bullae that may rupture.

PSORIASIS CH

Skin integrity, impaired may be related to increased epidermal cell proliferation and absence of normal protective skin layers possibly evidenced by scaling papules and plaques.

Body image disturbance may be related to cosmetically unsightly skin lesions possibly evidenced by hiding affected body part, negative feelings about body, feelings of helplessness, and change in social involvement.

PULMONARY EMBOLUS MS

Breathing pattern, ineffective may be related to tracheobronchial obstruction by inflammation, copious secretions or active bleeding; decreased lung expansion possibly evidenced by changes in depth and/or rate of respiration, dyspnea/use of accessory muscles, altered chest excursion, abnormal breath

---

*Note: A potential diagnosis is not evidenced by signs and symptoms as the problem has not occurred and nursing interventions are directed at prevention.

sounds (crackles, wheezes), and cough (with or without sputum production).

Gas exchange, impaired may be related to altered blood flow to alveoli or to major portions of the lung, altered oxygen supply (atelectasis, airway/alveolar collapse), and exchange problems (pulmonary edema/effusion, excessive secretions/active bleeding) possibly evidenced by profound dyspnea, restlessness, apprehension, somnolence, cyanosis, and changes in ABGs (hypoxemia and hypercapnea).

Tissue perfusion, altered, cardiopulmonary may be related to interruption of blood flow (arterial/venous), exchange problems at alveolar level, or at tissue level (acidotic shifting of the oxyhemoglobin curve) possibly evidenced by radiology/laboratory evidence of ventilation/perfusion mismatch, dyspnea, and central cyanosis.

Fear/Anxiety (specify level) may be related to severe dyspnea/inability to breathe normally, perceived threat of death, threat to/change in health status, physiologic response to hypoxemia/acidosis, and concern regarding unknown outcome of situation possibly evidenced by restlessness, irritability, withdrawal or attack behavior, sympathetic stimulation (cardiovascular excitation, pupil dilation, sweating, vomiting, diarrhea), crying, and voice quivering.

PURPURA, IDIOPATHIC THROMBOCYTOPENIA CH

*Injury, potential for** may be related to abnormal blood profile/risk of hemorrhage.

Activity intolerance may be related to decreased

---

*Note: A potential diagnosis is not evidenced by signs and symptoms as the problem has not occurred and nursing interventions are directed at prevention.

oxygen-carrying capacity/imbalance between oxygen supply and demand possibly evidenced by reports of fatigue/weakness.

Knowledge deficit [learning need] may be related to lack of information regarding therapy choices, outcomes, and self-care needs possibly evidenced by statements of concern, questions, and misconceptions.

PYELONEPHRITIS MS

Pain may be related to acute inflammation of renal tissues possibly evidenced by complaints (specify), guarding/distraction behaviors, self-focus, and autonomic responses (changes in vital signs).

Hyperthermia may be related to inflammatory process/increased metabolic rate possibly evidenced by increase in body temperature, warm/flushed skin, tachycardia, and chills.

Urinary elimination, altered patterns may be related to inflammation/irritation of bladder mucosa possibly evidenced by dysuria, urgency, and frequency.

Knowledge deficit [learning need] may be related to lack of information regarding therapy needs and prevention possibly evidenced by statements of concern, questions, and recurrence of condition.

■ Q

QUADRIPLEGIA,
(Refer Also to Paraplegia) MS

Breathing pattern, ineffective may be related to neuromuscular impairment possibly evidenced by decreased respiratory depth, dyspnea, cyanosis, and abnormal ABGs.

Grieving, anticipatory may be related to perceived loss of self, anticipated alterations in lifestyle and expectations, and limitation of future options/

choices possibly evidenced by expressions of distress, anger, and sorrow; choked feelings; and changes in eating habits, sleep, and communication patterns.

Self-care deficit, all areas related to neuromuscular impairment evidenced by inability to perform self-care tasks.

Home maintenance management, impaired may be related to permanent effects of injury, inadequate/absence of support systems and finances, and lack of familiarity with resources possibly evidenced by expressions of difficulties, requests for information and assistance, outstanding debts/financial crisis, and lack of necessary aides and equipment.

■ R

RABIES (EXPOSURE TO) — CH

*Infection, potential for** may be related to break in skin and exposure to rabies virus.

Knowledge deficit [learning need] may be related to lack of information regarding pathophysiology of infection, prophylaxis, and treatment needs possibly evidenced by statements of concern, questions, and misconceptions.

*Injury, potential for community health** may be related to presence of transmissible infectious disease (rabies) in wild and/or domesticated animals.

RAPE — PSY

Knowledge deficit [learning need] may be related to lack of information regarding prophylactic treat-

---

*Note: A potential diagnosis is not evidenced by signs and symptoms as the problem has not occurred and nursing interventions are directed at prevention.

ment for individual concerns (sexually transmitted diseases, pregnancy, required medical/legal procedures, community resources/supports) possibly evidenced by statements of concerns, questions, misconceptions, and exacerbation of symptoms.

Rape-trauma response (acute phase) related to actual or attempted sexual attack without consent possibly evidenced by wide range of emotional reactions, including anxiety, fear, anger, embarrassment, and multisystem physical complaints.

*Tissue integrity, impaired, potential** may be related to forceful sexual penetration and trauma to fragile tissues.

RAYNAUD'S DISEASE CH

Pain may be related to vasospasm/altered perfusion of affected tissues and ischemia/destruction of tissues possibly evidenced by verbal complaints, guarding of affected parts, self-focusing, and restlessness.

Tissue perfusion, altered, peripheral may be related to periodic reduction of arterial blood flow to affected areas possibly evidenced by pallor, cyanosis, numbness,, and paresthesia.

Knowledge deficit [learning need] may be related to lack of information regarding pathophysiology of the condition, potential for complications, therapy/self-care needs possibly evidenced by statements of concern, questions, and misconceptions.

REFLEX SYMPATHETIC DYSTROPHY (RSD) CH

Pain, (acute or) chronic may be related to continued nerve stimulation possibly evidenced by com-

---

*Note: A potential diagnosis is not evidenced by signs and symptoms as the problem has not occurred and nursing interventions are directed at prevention.

plaints (specify), distraction/guarding behaviors, narrowed focus, changes in sleep patterns, and altered ability to continue previous activities.

Tissue perfusion, altered, peripheral may be related to reduction of arterial blood flow (arteriole vasoconstriction) possibly evidenced by complaints of pain, decreased skin temperature and pallor, diminished arterial pulsations, and swelling.

Sensory-perceptual alteration, tactile may be related to altered sensory reception possibly evidenced by change in usual response to stimuli/abnormal sensitivity of touch, physiologic anxiety, and irritability.

*Role performance, altered, potential** may be related to situational crisis and chronic disability.

*Family coping, compromised, potential** may be related to temporary family disorganization and role changes and prolonged disability that exhausts the supportive capacity of significant other(s).

RENAL FAILURE MS

Fluid volume, excess may be related to compromised regulatory mechanisms (decreased kidney function) possibly evidenced by weight gain, edema/anasarca, intake greater than output, venous congestion, and altered electrolyte levels.

Nutrition, altered: Less than body requirements may be related to inability to ingest/digest adequate nutrients (anorexia, nausea/vomiting, and ulcerations of oral mucosa) in addition to therapeutic dietary restrictions possibly evidenced by weight loss/loss of muscle mass, lack of interest in food/aversion to eating, and observed inadequate intake.

---

*Note: A potential diagnosis is not evidenced by signs and symptoms as the problem has not occurred and nursing interventions are directed at prevention.

*Infection, potential for** may be related to depression of immunologic defenses, invasive procedures, and malnutrition.

Thought processes, altered may be related to accumulation of toxic waste products and altered cerebral perfusion possibly evidenced by disorientation, changes in recent memory, apathy, and episodic obtundation.

Fatigue may be related to decreased metabolic energy production/dietary restrictions, anemia, increased energy requirements, e.g., fever/inflammation and tissue regeneration possibly evidenced by overwhelming lack of energy, inability to maintain usual activities, decreased performance, lethargy, and disinterest in surroundings.

Adjustment, impaired may be related to disability requiring change in lifestyle, inadequate support systems, and altered locus of control possibly evidenced by verbalization of nonacceptance of health status change, lack of movement toward independence, extended period of shock, disbelief, or anger regarding health status change, and lack of future-oriented thinking.

RENAL TRANSPLANTATION MS

*Fluid volume, excess, potential** may be related to compromised regulatory mechanism (implantation of new kidney requiring adjustment period for optimal functioning).

Body image disturbance may be related to failure and subsequent replacement of body part and medication-induced changes in appearance possibly evidenced by preoccupation with loss/change, hiding body part(s), negative feelings and changes in social involvement.

---

*Note: A potential diagnosis is not evidenced by signs and symptoms as the problem has not occurred and nursing interventions are directed at prevention.

Fear may be related to potential for transplant rejection/failure and threat of death possibly evidenced by increased tension, apprehension, concentration on source and verbalizations of concern.

*Infection, potential for** may be related to broken skin/traumatized tissue, stasis of body fluids, immunosuppression, invasive procedures, and chronic disease.

RESPIRATORY DISTRESS SYNDROME, NEWBORN

(Refer Also to Neonatal, Premature Newborn.) **PED/OB**

Gas exchange, impaired may be related to alveolar-capillary membrane changes (inadequate surfactant levels), altered oxygen supply (tracheobronchial obstruction, atelectasis), altered blood flow (immaturity of pulmonary arteriole musculature), altered oxygen-carrying capacity of blood (anemia) possibly evidenced by tachypnea, use of accessory muscles, retractions, expiratory grunting, pallor or cyanosis, abnormal ABGs, and tachycardia.

*Infection, potential for** may be related to inadequate primary defenses (decreased ciliary action, stasis of body fluids, traumatized tissues), inadequate secondary defenses (deficiency of neutrophils and specific immunoglobulins), invasive procedures, and malnutrition (absence of nutrient stores, increased metabolic demands).

*Tissue perfusion, altered, gastrointestinal, potential** may be related to persistent fetal circulation and tissue hypoxia/ischemia.

Parenting, altered, actual or potential [bonding] may be related to interruption/postponement of

---

*Note: A potential diagnosis is not evidenced by signs and symptoms as the problem has not occurred and nursing interventions are directed at prevention.

bonding process and separation from infant possibly evidenced by lack of parental attachment behaviors.

RETINAL DETACHMENT MS/CH

Sensory-perceptual alterations, visual related to decreased sensory reception possibly evidenced by visual distortions, decreased visual field, and changes in visual acuity.

Knowledge deficit [learning need] may be related to lack of information regarding therapy, prognosis, and self-care needs possibly evidenced by statements of concern and questions.

*Home maintenance management, impaired, potential** may be related to postoperative activity restrictions/limitations.

REYE'S SYNDROME PED

Fluid volume deficit (1 and 2) may be related to failure of regulatory mechanism (diabetes insipidus), excessive gastric losses (pernicious vomiting), and altered intake possibly evidenced by increased/dilute urine output, sudden weight loss, decreased venous filling, dry mucous membranes, decreased skin turgor, hypotension, and tachycardia.

Tissue perfusion, decreased cerebral may be related to diminished arterial/venous blood flow, and hypovolemia, possibly evidenced by memory loss, altered consciousness, and restlessness/agitation.

*Trauma, potential for** may be related to generalized weakness, reduced coordination, and cognitive deficits.

Breathing pattern, ineffective may be related to

---

*Note: A potential diagnosis is not evidenced by signs and symptoms as the problem has not occurred and nursing interventions are directed at prevention.

decreased energy and fatigue, cognitive impairment, tracheobronchial obstruction, and inflammatory process (aspiration pneumonia) possibly evidenced by tachypnea, abnormal ABGs, cough, and use of accessory muscles.

RHEUMATIC FEVER PED

Pain may be related to migratory inflammation of joints possibly evidenced by complaints (specify), guarding/distraction behaviors, self-focus, and autonomic responses (changes in vital signs).

Hyperthermia may be related to inflammatory process/hypermetabolic state possibly evidenced by increased body temperature, warm/flushed skin, and tachycardia.

Activity intolerance may be related to generalized weakness, joint pain, and medical restrictions/bedrest possibly evidenced by reports of fatigue, exertional discomfort, and abnormal heart rate in response to activity.

*Cardiac output, decreased, potential** may be related to cardiac inflammation/enlargement and altered contractility.

RICKETS (OSTEOMALACIA) PED

Growth and development, altered may be related to dietary deficiencies/indiscretions, malabsorption syndrome, and lack of exposure to sunlight possibly evidenced by altered physical growth and delay or difficulty in performing motor skills typical for age.

Knowledge deficit [learning need] may be related to lack of information regarding cause, pathophysiology, and therapy needs/prevention possibly evidenced by statements of concern, questions, mis-

---

*Note: A potential diagnosis is not evidenced by signs and symptoms as the problem has not occurred and nursing interventions are directed at prevention.

conceptions, and inaccurate follow-through of instructions.

RINGWORM, TINEA

(Refer Also to Athlete's foot) **CH**

Skin integrity, impaired may be related to fungal infection of the dermis possibly evidenced by disruption of skin surfaces/presence of lesions.

Knowledge deficit [learning need] may be related to lack of information regarding infectious nature, therapy, and self-care needs possibly evidenced by statements of concern, questions, and recurrence/spread.

RUBELLA **PED**

Pain may be related to inflammatory effects of viral infection and presence of desquamating rash possibly evidenced by complaints (specify), distraction behaviors/restlessness.

Knowledge deficit [learning need] may be related to lack of information regarding contagious nature, possible complications, and self-care needs possibly evidenced by statements of concern, questions, and inaccurate follow-through of instructions.

■ S

SCABIES **CH**

Skin integrity, impaired may be related to presence of invasive parasite and development of pruritus possibly evidenced by disruption of skin surface and inflammation.

Knowledge deficit [learning need] may be related to lack of information regarding communicable nature, possible complications, therapy, and self-care needs possibly evidenced by questions and statements of concern about spread to others.

SCARLET FEVER PED

Hyperthermia may be related to effects of circulating toxins possibly evidenced by increased body temperature, warm/flushed skin, and tachycardia.

Pain (discomfort) may be related to inflammation of mucous membranes and effects of circulating toxins (malaise, fever) possibly evidenced by complaints (specify), distraction behaviors, guarding (decreased swallowing), and self-focus.

*Fluid volume deficit, potential** may be related to hypermetabolic state (hyperthermia) and reduced intake.

SCHIZOPHRENIC DISORDERS PSY

Thought process, altered may be related to presence of psychologic conflicts possibly evidenced by impaired ability to reason/problem solve, inappropriate affect, delusions, and auditory hallucinations.

Social isolation may be related to alterations in mental status, unacceptable social behaviors, inadequate personal resources, and inability to engage in satisfying personal relationships possibly evidenced by dull affect, uncommunicative/withdrawn behavior, seeking, to be alone, and inadequate or absence of significant purpose in life.

Health maintenance management, altered may be related to altered ability to make deliberate and thoughtful judgments, altered communications, and possible lack of material resources possibly evidenced by inability to take responsibility for meeting basic health practices in any or all functional areas and demonstrated lack of adaptive behaviors to internal or external environmental changes.

*Violence, potential for, directed at self/others**

---

*Note: A potential diagnosis is not evidenced by signs and symptoms as the problem has not occurred and nursing interventions are directed at prevention.

may be related to disturbances of thinking/feeling (depression, paranoia, suicidal ideation).

Coping, ineffective, individual **may be related to personal vulnerability, inadequate support system(s), unrealistic perceptions, inadequate coping methods, and disintegration of thought processes possibly evidenced by impaired judgment/cognition and perception, diminished problem-solving/decision-making capacities, poor self-esteem, chronic anxiety, depression, inability to perform role expectations, and alteration in social participation.**

Family coping, disabling **may be related to ambivalent family system/relationships and difficulty of family members in coping effectively with patient's maladaptive behaviors possibly evidenced by patient's expressions of despair at family's lack of reaction/involvement, neglectful relationships with patient, extreme distortion regarding patient's health problem including extreme denial about its existence/severity or prolonged overconcern, impaired restructuring of a meaningful life for individual family members, and impaired individuation.**

Self-care deficit, (specify) **may be related to perceptual and cognitive impairment, immobility (withdrawal/isolation and decreased psychomotor activity), and side effects of psychotropic medications possibly evidenced by inability to/or difficulty in areas of feeding self, keeping body clean, dressing appropriately and/or toileting self, and changes in bowel/bladder elimination.**

SCIATICA CH

Pain **may be related to peripheral nerve root compression possibly evidenced by complaints**

***Note: A potential diagnosis is not evidenced by signs and symptoms as the problem has not occurred and nursing interventions are directed at prevention.**

(specify), guarding/distraction behaviors, and self-focus.

Mobility, impaired physical may be related to neurologic pain and muscular involvement possibly evidenced by reluctance to attempt movement and decreased muscle strength/mass.

SCLERODERMA

(Refer also to Lupus Erythematosus, systemic) **CH**

Mobility, impaired physical may be related to musculoskeletal impairment and associated pain possibly evidenced by decreased strength, decreased range of motion, and reluctance to attempt movement.

Tissue perfusion, altered, (specify) may be related to reduced arterial blood flow (arteriolar vasoconstriction) possibly evidenced by changes in skin temperature/color, ulcer formation, and changes in organ function (cardiopulmonary, gastrointestinal, renal).

Nutrition, altered: Less than body requirements may be related to inability to ingest/digest/absorb adequate nutrients (sclerosis of the tissues rendering mouth immobile, decreased peristalsis of esophagus and small intestines, atrophy of smooth muscle of colon) possibly evidenced by weight loss, decreased intake, inability to ingest food, and reported/observed difficulty swallowing.

Adjustment, impaired may be related to disability requiring change in lifestyle, inadequate support systems, assault to self-esteem, and altered locus of control possibly evidenced by verbalization of nonacceptance of health status change and lack of

---

*Note: A potential diagnosis is not evidenced by signs and symptoms as the problem has not occurred and nursing interventions are directed at prevention.

movement toward independence/future-oriented thinking.

Body image disturbance may be related to skin changes with induration, atrophy, and fibrosis, loss of hair, and skin and muscle contractures possibly evidenced by verbalization of negative feelings about body, focus on past strength/function or appearance, fear of rejection or of reaction by others, hiding body part, and change in social involvement.

SCOLIOSIS PED

Body image disturbance may be related to altered body structure, use of therapeutic device(s), and activity restrictions possibly evidenced by negative feelings about body, change in social involvement and preoccupation with situation or refusal to acknowledge problem.

Knowledge deficit [learning need] may be related to lack of information regarding pathophysiology of condition and therapy needs and outcomes possibly evidenced by statements of concern, questions, misconceptions, and inaccurate follow-through of instructions.

Adjustment, impaired may be related to lack of comprehension of long-term consequences of behavior possibly evidenced by failure to adhere to treatment regimen/keep appointments and evidence of failure to improve.

SEBORRHEIC DERMATITIS CH

Skin integrity, impaired may be related to chronic inflammatory condition of the skin possibly evidenced by disruption of skin surface with dry or

---

*Note: A potential diagnosis is not evidenced by signs and symptoms as the problem has not occurred and nursing interventions are directed at prevention.

moist scales, yellowish crusts, erythema, and fissures.

SEPSIS, PUERPERAL OB

*Infection, potential for spread/septic shock** may be related to broken skin, traumatized tissues, stasis of body fluids, invasive procedures, and altered immune response.

Hyperthermia may be related to inflammatory process/hypermetabolic state possibly evidenced by increase in body temperature, warm/flushed skin, and tachycardia.

Parenting, altered, actual/potential may be related to presence of physical illness, medical/therapeutic interruption in bonding process, and threat to own survival possibly evidenced by incomplete parental attachment behaviors and verbalized concern regarding role inadequacy.

*Tissue perfusion, altered, peripheral, potential** may be related to interruption/reduction of blood flow (presence of infectious thrombi).

SEPTICEMIA

(Refer Also to Sepsis) MS

Tissue perfusion, altered, (specify) may be related to changes in arterial/venous blood flow (selective vasoconstriction, presence of microemboli) and hypovolemia possibly evidenced by changes in skin temperature/color, changes in blood pressure and pulse pressure, changes in sensorium, and decreased urinary output.

*Fluid volume deficit, potential** may be related to presence of hypermetabolic state, vascular shifts to interstitial space, and reduced intake.

*Cardiac output, decreased, potential** may be re-

---

*Note: A potential diagnosis is not evidenced by signs and symptoms as the problem has not occurred and nursing interventions are directed at prevention.

lated to decreased preload (venous return and circulating volume), altered afterload (increased systemic vascular resistance), negative inotropic effects of hypoxia, complement activation, and lysosomal hydrolase.

SERUM SICKNESS CH

Pain may be related to inflammation of the joints and skin eruptions possibly evidenced by complaints (specify), guarding/distraction behaviors, and self-focus.

Knowledge deficit [learning need] may be related to lack of information regarding nature of condition, treatment needs, potential complications, and need to avoid causative agent possibly evidenced by statements of concern, questions, and inaccurate follow-through of instructions.

SEXUALLY TRANSMITTED DISEASE CH

*Infection, potential for transmission** may be related to contagious nature of infecting agent and insufficient knowledge to avoid exposure to/transmission of pathogens.

Skin/Tissue integrity, impaired may be related to invasion of/irritation by pathogenic organism(s) possibly evidenced by disruptions of skin and inflammation of mucous membranes.

Knowledge deficit [learning need] may be related to lack of information regarding pathophysiology of condition, outcomes/complications, therapy needs, and transmission possibly evidenced by statements of concern, questions, misconceptions, and inaccurate follow-through of instructions.

---

*Note: A potential diagnosis is not evidenced by signs and symptoms as the problem has not occurred and nursing interventions are directed at prevention.

SHOCK

(Refer Also to Shock, Cardiogenic and Hemorrhagic) **MS**

Tissue perfusion, altered, (specify) may be related to changes in circulating volume and/or vascular tone possibly evidenced by changes in skin color/temperature and pulse pressure, reduced blood pressure, changes in mentation, and decreased urinary output.

Anxiety (specify level) may be related to change in health status and threat of death possibly evidenced by increased tension, apprehension, sympathetic stimulation, restlessness, and expressions of concern.

SHOCK, CARDIOGENIC **MS**

Cardiac output, decreased may be related to structural damage, decreased myocardial contractility, and presence of dysrhythmias possibly evidenced by ECG changes, variations in hemodynamic readings, jugular vein distention, cold/clammy skin, diminished peripheral pulses, and decreased urinary output.

SHOCK, HEMORRHAGIC **MS**

Fluid volume deficit, (2) [active loss] may be related to excessive vascular loss possibly evidenced by hypotension, tachycardia, decreased pulse volume and pressure, change in mentation, and decreased/concentrated urine.

SICK SINUS SYNDROME **MS**

Cardiac output, decreased may be related to alterations in rate, rhythm, and electrical conduction possibly evidenced by ECG evidence of dysrhythmias, complaints of palpitations/weakness, changes in mentation/consciousness, and syncope.

*Trauma, potential for** may be related to changes

---

*See footnote on preceding page.

in cerebral perfusion with altered consciousness/loss of balance.

SNOW BLINDNESS CH

Sensory-perceptual alteration, visual may be related to altered status of sense organ (irritation of the conjunctiva, hyperemia) possibly evidenced by intolerance to light (photophobia) and decreased/loss of visual acuity.

Pain may be related to irritation/vascular congestion of the conjunctiva possibly evidenced by complaints (specify), guarding/distraction behaviors and self-focus.

Anxiety (specify level) may be related to situational crisis and threat to/change in health status possibly evidenced by increased tension, apprehension, uncertainty, worry, restlessness, and focus on self.

SOMATOFORM DISORDERS PSY

*Violence, potential for self-directed** may be related to depressed mood, feelings of powerlessness over physical condition, belief that s/he has a serious illness, and hysterical response to chronic pain.

Pain, chronic may be related to severe level of anxiety, repressed/low self-esteem, unmet dependency needs, history of self or loved one having experienced a serious illness, fixation in earlier level of development, retarded ego development, and inadequate coping skills possibly evidenced by multiple somatic complaints of several years' duration, absence of physiologic evidence for physical symptoms, narcissistic tendencies with total focus on self and physical symptoms, demanding behav-

---

*Note: A potential diagnosis is not evidenced by signs and symptoms as the problem has not occurred and nursing interventions are directed at prevention.

iors, and denial of correlation between physical symptoms and psychologic problems.

Coping, ineffective, individual may be related to severe level of anxiety that is repressed/low self-esteem, unmet dependency needs, fixation in earlier level of development, retarded ego development, and inadequate coping skills possibly evidenced by multiple somatic complaints of several years' duration, demanding behaviors, and refusal to attend therapeutic activities.

Social isolation may be related to severe level of anxiety, low self-esteem, preoccupation with self and physical symptoms, chronic pain, and rejection by others due to focus on self/physical symptoms possibly evidenced by sad/dull affect, absence of supportive significant other(s), uncommunicative/withdrawn behavior, lack of eye contact, and seeking to be alone.

SPRAIN, ANKLE CH

Pain may be related to trauma to/swelling in joint possibly evidenced by complaints (specify), guarding/distraction behaviors, self-focusing, and autonomic responses (changes in vital signs).

Mobility, impaired physical may be related to musculoskeletal injury, pain, and therapeutic restrictions possibly evidenced by reluctance to attempt movement and limited range of motion.

STAPEDECTOMY MS

*Trauma, potential for** may be related to increased middle-ear pressure with displacement of prosthesis and balancing difficulties/dizziness.

*Infection, potential for** may be related to surgi-

---

*Note: A potential diagnosis is not evidenced by signs and symptoms as the problem has not occurred and nursing interventions are directed at prevention.

cally traumatized tissue, invasive procedures, and environmental exposure to upper respiratory infections.

Pain may be related to surgical trauma, edema formation, and presence of packing possibly evidenced by complaints (specify), guarding/distraction behaviors, and self-focus.

SUBSTANCE DEPENDENCY/ABUSE

(Refer Also to Poisoning, Drug) **PSY**

Coping, ineffective, individual may be related to personal vulnerability, difficulty handling new situations, previous ineffective/inadequate coping skills with substitution of drug(s), and anxiety/fear possibly evidenced by denial, lack of acceptance that drug use is causing the present situation, altered social patterns/participation, impaired adaptive behavior and problem-solving skills, and decreased ability to handle stress of illness/hospitalization.

Powerlessness may be related to substance addiction with/without periods of abstinence, episodic compulsive indulgence, attempts at recovery, and lifestyle of helplessness possibly evidenced by ineffective recovery attempts, continuous/constant thinking about drug and/or obtaining drug, alteration in personal/occupational and social life.

Family, coping, compromised/dysfunctional may be related to personal vulnerability of individual family members, co-dependency issues, situational crises, compromised social systems, family disorganization/role changes, and prolonged disease progression that exhausts supportive capability of family members possibly evidenced by denial, lack of acceptance that drinking/drug use is causing the present situation, or belief that all problems are due to substance use, severely dysfunctional family (e.g., family violence, spouse/child abuse, separation/divorce), financial affairs in disarray, and employment difficulties.

Sexual dysfunction may be related to altered body function (neurologic damage and debilitating effects of drug use) possibly evidenced by progressive interference with sexual functioning; a significant degree of testicular atrophy, gynecomastia, impotence/decreased sperm counts in men; and loss of body hair, thin/soft skin, spider angioma, and amenorrhea/increase in miscarriages in women.

SURGERY, GENERAL MS

Anxiety (specify level) Fear may be related to change in health status and threat of death and to self-concept possibly evidenced by increased tension, apprehension, fear of unspecific consequences, sympathetic stimulation, and restlessness.

Knowledge deficit [learning need] may be related to lack of information regarding surgical procedure/expectation, postoperative routines/therapy, and self-care needs possibly evidenced by statements of concern, questions, and misconceptions.

*Breathing pattern, ineffective, potential** may be related to chemically induced muscular relaxation, perception/cognitive impairment, decreased energy, and incisional pain.

*Fluid volume deficit, potential** may be related to preoperative/postoperative fluid deprivation, blood loss, and excessive GI losses (vomiting).

Pain may be related to intraoperative positioning, muscle retractions, and tissue trauma/presence of incision possibly evidenced by complaints (specify), guarding/distraction behaviors, self-focus, and autonomic responses (changes in vital signs).

---

*Note: A potential diagnosis is not evidenced by signs and symptoms as the problem has not occurred and nursing interventions are directed at prevention.

SYNOVITIS (KNEE) CH

Pain may be related to inflammation of synovial membrane of the joint with effusion possibly evidenced by complaints (specify), guarding/distraction behaviors, self-focus, and autonomic responses, (changes in vital signs).

Mobility impaired, physical may be related to pain and decreased strength of joint possibly evidenced by limited range of motion and reluctance to attempt movement.

SYPHILIS, CONGENITAL (Refer Also to Sexually Transmitted Disease) PED

Pain may be related to inflammatory process, edema formation, and development of skin lesions possibly evidenced by irritability/crying that may be increased with movement of extremities and autonomic responses (changes in vital signs).

Skin/Tissue integrity, impaired may be related to development of lesions/rash and irritation of mucous membranes possibly evidenced by disruption of skin surfaces and rhinitis.

Growth and development, altered may be related to effects of infectious process possibly evidenced by altered physical growth and delay or difficulty performing skills typical of age group.

Knowledge deficit [learning need] may be related to caretaker/parental lack of information regarding pathophysiology of condition, transmissibility, therapy needs, expected outcomes, and potential complications possibly evidenced by statements of concern, questions, and misconceptions.

SYRINGOMYELIA MS

Sensory-perceptual alterations, (specify) may be related to neurologic lesion altering sensory reception possibly evidenced by change in usual response to stimuli and motor incoordination.

Anxiety (specify level)/Fear may be related to change in health status, threat of change in role functioning and socioeconomic status, and threat to self-concept possibly evidenced by increased tension, apprehension, uncertainty, focus on self, and expressed concerns.

Mobility, impaired physical may be related to neuromuscular and sensory impairment possibly evidenced by decreased muscle strength, control and mass, and impaired coordination.

Self-care deficit, (specify) may be related to neuromuscular and sensory impairments possibly evidenced by statements of inability to perform care tasks.

■ T

TAY-SACHS DISEASE PED

Growth and development, altered may be related to effects of physical condition possibly evidenced by altered physical growth, loss of/failure to acquire skills typical of age, flat affect, and decreased responses.

Sensory-perceptual alterations, visual may be related to neurologic deterioration of optic nerve possibly evidenced by loss of visual acuity.

Grieving, anticipatory (family) may be related to expected eventual loss of infant possibly evidenced by expressions of distress, denial, guilt, anger, and sorrow; choked feelings; changes in sleep/eating habits; and altered libido.

Powerlessness (family) may be related to absence of therapeutic interventions for progressive/fatal disease possibly evidenced by verbal expressions of having no control over situation/outcome and depression over physical/mental deterioration.

*Spiritual distress, potential** may be related to

---

*See footnote on following page.

challenged belief and value system by presence of fatal condition with racial/religious connotations and intense suffering.

Family coping, compromised may be related to situational crisis, temporary preoccupation with managing emotional conflicts and personal suffering, family disorganization, and prolonged/progressive disease possibly evidenced by preoccupations with personal reactions, expressed concern about reactions of other family members, inadequate support of one another and altered communication patterns.

THROMBOPHLEBITIS MS

Tissue perfusion, altered, peripheral may be related to interruption of venous blood flow possibly evidenced by changes in skin color/temperature over affected area and development of edema.

Pain may be related to vascular inflammation/irritation and edema formation possibly evidenced by complaints (specify), guarding/distraction behaviors, and self-focus.

Knowledge deficit [learning need] may be related to lack of information regarding pathophysiology of condition, therapy/self-care needs and possibility of embolization possibly evidenced by statements of concern, questions, inaccurate follow-through of instructions, and development of preventable complications.

CH

*Mobility, impaired physical, potential** may be related to pain and discomfort and restrictive therapies/safety precautions.

---

*Note: A potential diagnosis is not evidenced by signs and symptoms as the problem has not occurred and nursing interventions are directed at prevention.

THROMBOSIS, DEEP VENOUS

(Refer to Thrombophlebitis) **MS**

THYROIDECTOMY

(Refer Also to Hyperthyroidism, Hypothyroidism, and Hypoparathyroidism) **MS**

*Airway clearance, ineffective, potential** may be related to hematoma/edema formation with tracheal obstruction.

*Trauma, potential for, to head/neck** may be related to loss of muscle control/support and position of suture line.

Pain may be related to presence of surgical incision and tissue trauma/edema possibly evidenced by complaints (specify), guarding/distraction behaviors, self-focus, and autonomic responses (changes in vital signs).

Communication, impaired verbal may be related to tissue edema, pain/discomfort, and vocal cord injury/laryngeal nerve damage possibly evidenced by impaired articulation, does not/cannot speak and use of nonverbal cues.

THYROTOXICOSIS

(Refer Also to Hyperthyroidism) **MS**

*Cardiac output, decreased, potential** may be related to uncontrolled hypermetabolic state increasing cardiac workload, changes in venous return and systemic vascular resistance, and alterations in rate, rhythm, and electrical conduction.

Anxiety (specify level) may be related to physiologic factors: hypermetabolic state (central nervous system stimulation) and pseudocatecholamine effect of thyroid hormones possibly evidenced by in-

---

*Note: A potential diagnosis is not evidenced by signs and symptoms as the problem has not occurred and nursing interventions are directed at prevention.

creased feelings of apprehension, shakiness, loss of control, panic, changes in cognition, distortion of environmental stimuli, extraneous movements, restlessness, and tremors.

*Thought processes, altered, potential** may be related to physiologic changes (increased central nervous system stimulation/accelerated mental activity), and altered sleep patterns.

Knowledge deficit [learning need] may be related to lack of information regarding effects of condition and treatment needs and potential for complications/crisis situation possibly evidenced by statements of concern, questions, misconceptions, and inaccurate follow-through of instructions.

TIC DOULOUREUX

(Refer to Trigeminal Neuralgia) **CH**

TONSILLECTOMY

(Refer to Adenoidectomy) **PED**

TONSILLITIS **PED**

Pain may be related to inflammation of tonsils and effects of circulating toxins possibly evidenced by complaints (specify), distraction behaviors, guarding (reluctance/refusal to swallow), self-focus, and autonomic responses (changes in vital signs).

Hyperthermia may be related to presence of inflammation process/hypermetabolic state, and dehydration possibly evidenced by increased body temperature, warm/flushed skin, and tachycardia.

Knowledge deficity [learning need] may be related to lack of information regarding cause/transmission, treatment needs, and potential complica-

---

*Note: A potential diagnosis is not evidenced by signs and symptoms as the problem has not occurred and nursing interventions are directed at prevention.

tions possibly evidenced by statements of concern, questions, inaccurate follow-through of instructions, and recurrence of condition.

TOTAL JOINT REPLACEMENT MS

*Infection, potential for** may be related to inadequate primary defenses (broken skin, exposure of joint), inadequate secondary defenses/immunosuppression (long-term corticosteroid use), invasive procedures, surgical manipulation, implantation of foreign body, and decreased mobility.

Mobility, impaired physical may be related to pain and discomfort, musculoskeletal impairment, and surgery/restrictive therapies possibly evidenced by reluctance to attempt movement, difficulty purposefully moving within the physical environment, complaints of pain/discomfort on movement, limited range of motion, and decreased muscle strength/control.

*Tissue perfusion, altered, peripheral, potential** may be related to reduced arterial/venous blood flow, direct trauma to blood vessels, tissue edema, improper location/dislocation of prosthesis, and hypovolemia.

Pain may be related to physical agents (traumatized tissues/surgical intervention, degeneration of joints) and psychologic factors (anxiety, advanced age) possibly evidenced by complaints (specify), distraction/guarding behaviors, self-focus, and autonomic responses (changes in vital signs).

TOXEMIA OF PREGNANCY

(Refer to Pregnancy-Induced Hypertension.) **OB**

---

*Note: A potential diagnosis is not evidenced by signs and symptoms as the problem has not occurred and nursing interventions are directed at prevention.

TOXIC SHOCK SYNDROME

(Refer Also to Septicemia.) **MS**

Hyperthermia may be related to inflammatory process/hypermetabolic state and dehydration possibly evidenced by increased body temperature, warm/flushed skin, and tachycardia.

Fluid volume deficit, (2) [active loss] may be related to increased gastric losses (diarrhea, vomiting), fever/hypermetabolic state, and decreased intake possibly evidenced by dry mucous membranes, increased pulse, hypotension, delayed venous filling, decreased/concentrated urine, and hemoconcentration.

Pain may be related to inflammatory process, effects of circulating toxins, and skin disruptions possibly evidenced by complaints (specify), guarding/distraction behaviors, self-focus, and autonomic responses (changes in vital signs).

Skin/Tissue integrity, impaired may be related to effects of circulating toxins and dehydration possibly evidenced by development of desquamating rash, hyperemia and inflammation of mucous membranes.

TRACTION **MS**

Pain may be related to direct trauma to tissue/bone and therapy restrictions possibly evidenced by complaints (specify), guarding/distraction behaviors, self-focus, and autonomic responses (changes in vital signs).

Mobility, impaired physical may be related to skeletal impairment, pain, and therapeutic restrictions of movement possibly evidenced by limited range of motion, inability to move purposefully in environment, and reluctance to attempt movement.

*Infection, potential for** may be related to inva-

---

*See footnote on following page.

sive procedures including insertion of foreign body through skin/bone, presence of traumatized tissue, and reduced activity with stasis of body fluids.

Diversional activity deficit may be related to length of hospitalization and environmental lack of usual activity possibly evidenced by statements of boredom, restlessness, and irritability.

TRICHINOSIS CH

Pain may be related to parasitic invasion of muscle tissues, edema of upper eyelids, small localized hemorrhages, and development of urticaria possibly evidenced by complaints (specify), guarding, distraction behaviors/restlessness, and autonomic responses (changes in vital signs).

Fluid volume deficit, (2) [active loss] may be related to hypermetabolic state (fever, diaphoresis), excessive gastric losses (vomiting, diarrhea), and decreased intake/difficulty swallowing possibly evidenced by dry mucous membranes, decreased skin turgor, hypotension, decreased venous filling, decreased/concentrated urine, and hemoconcentration.

Breathing pattern, ineffective may be related to myositis of the diaphragm and intercostal muscles possibly evidenced by resulting changes in respiratory depth, tachypnea, dyspnea, and abnormal arterial blood gases.

Knowledge deficit [learning need] may be related to lack of information regarding cause/prevention of condition, therapy needs, and possible complications possibly evidenced by statements of concern, questions, and misconceptions.

---

*Note: A potential diagnosis is not evidenced by signs and symptoms as the problem has not occurred and nursing interventions are directed at prevention.

TUBERCULOSIS (PULMONARY) CH

*Infection, potential for spread/reactivation** may be related to inadequate primary defenses (decreased ciliary action/stasis of secretions, tissue destruction/extension of infection), lowered resistance/suppressed inflammatory response, malnutrition, environmental exposure, and insufficient knowledge to avoid exposure to pathogens.

Airway clearance, ineffective may be related to thick, viscous or bloody secretions, fatigue/poor cough effort, and tracheal/pharyngeal edema possibly evidenced by abnormal respiratory rate, rhythm, and depth and abnormal breath sounds (rhonchi, wheezes), stridor and dyspnea.

*Gas exchange, impaired, potential** may be related to decrease in effective lung surface, atelectasis, destruction of alveolar-capillary membrane and bronchial edema.

Activity intolerance may be related to imbalance between oxygen supply and demand possibly evidenced by reports of fatigue, weakness, and exertional dyspnea.

Nutrition, altered: Less than body requirements may be related to inability to ingest adequate nutrients (anorexia, effects of drug therapy, fatigue, insufficient financial resources) possibly evidenced by weight loss, reported lack of interest in food/altered taste sensation, and poor muscle tone.

*Noncompliance (specify) [compliance, altered] potential** may be related to lengthy therapy requirements even after remission of symptoms as well as side effects of therapy.

---

*Note: A potential diagnosis is not evidenced by signs and symptoms as the problem has not occurred and nursing interventions are directed at prevention.

TYMPANOPLASTY

(Refer to Stapedectomy.) **MS**

TYPHUS (TICK-BORNE/ROCKY MOUNTAIN SPOTTED FEVER) **MS**

Hyperthermia may be related to generalized inflammatory process (vasculitis) possibly evidenced by increased body temperature, warm/flushed skin, and tachycardia.

Pain may be related to generalized vasculitis and edema formation possibly evidenced by complaints (specify), guarding/distraction behaviors, self-focus, and autonomic responses (changes in vital signs).

Tissue perfusion, altered, (specify) may be related to reduction/interruption of blood flow (generalized vasculitis/thrombi formation) possibly evidenced by complaints of headache/abdominal pain, changes in mentation, and areas of peripheral ulceration/necrosis.

■ U

ULCER, DECUBITUS **MS/CH**

Skin/Tissue integrity, impaired may be related to altered circulation, nutritional deficit, fluid imbalance, impaired physical mobility, irritation of body excretions/secretions, and sensory impairments evidenced by tissue damage/destruction.

Pain may be related to destruction of protective skin layers and exposure of nerves possibly evidenced by complaints (specify), distraction behaviors, and self-focus.

*Infection, potential for** may be related to bro-

---

*Note: A potential diagnosis is not evidenced by signs and symptoms as the problem has not occurred and nursing interventions are directed at prevention.

ken/traumatized tissue and increased environmental exposure, and nutritional deficits.

ULCER, PEPTIC MS/CH

Fluid volume deficit, (2) [active loss] may be related to vascular losses (hemorrhage) possibly evidenced by hypotension, tachycardia, delayed capillary refill, changes in mentation, restlessness, concentrated/decreased urine, pallor, and diaphoresis.

*Tissue perfusion, altered, (specify), potential** may be related to hypovolemia.

Fear/Anxiety (specify level) may be related to change in health status and threat of death possibly evidenced by increased tension, restlessness, irritability, fearfulness, trembling, tachycardia, diaphoresis, lack of eye contact, focus on self, withdrawal, and panic or attack behavior.

Pain may be related to caustic irritation/destruction of gastric tissues possibly evidenced by complaints (specify), distraction behaviors, self-focus, and autonomic responses (changes in vital signs).

Knowledge deficit [learning need] may be related to lack of information regarding pathophysiology of condition, therapy/self-care needs, and potential complications possibly evidenced by statements of concern, questions, inaccurate follow-through of instructions, and recurrence of condition.

ULCER, PRESSURE

(Refer to Ulcer, Decubitus) CH

Tissue perfusion, altered, peripheral may be related to reduced/interrupted blood flow possibly evidenced by presence of inflamed, necrotic lesion.

---

*Note: A potential diagnosis is not evidenced by signs and symptoms as the problem has not occurred and nursing interventions are directed at prevention.

Knowledge deficit [learning need] may be related to lack of information regarding cause and prevention of condition and potential complications possibly evidenced by statements of concern, questions, misconceptions, and inaccurate follow-through of instructions.

UNCONSCIOUSNESS (COMA) MS

*Suffocation, potential for** may be related to cognitive impairment/loss of protective reflexes and purposeful movement.

*Trauma, potential for** may be related to cognitive impairment, generalized weakness/reduced coordination, and absence of purposeful movement.

Self-care deficit, total may be related to cognitive impairment and absence of purposeful activity possibly evidenced by inability to perform tasks of care.

*Tissue perfusion, altered, cerebral, potential** may be related to reduced/interrupted arterial/venous blood flow (direct injury, edema formation).

*Infection, potential for** may be related to stasis of body fluids (oral, pulmonary, urinary), invasive procedures, and nutritional deficits.

URINARY DIVERSION CH

*Skin integrity, impaired, potential** may be related to absence of sphincter at stoma, character/flow of urine from stoma, reaction to product/chemicals, and improper fitting of appliance or removal of adhesive.

*Body image/Self-esteem, disturbance, potential** may be related to biophysical factors: presence of stoma, loss of control of urine elimination; and psy-

---

*Note: A potential diagnosis is not evidenced by signs and symptoms as the problem has not occurred and nursing interventions are directed at prevention.

chosocial factors: altered body structure, disease process, and associated treatment regimen (cancer).

Pain may be related to physical factors: disruption of skin/tissues (incisions/drains); biologic: activity of disease process (cancer, trauma); psychologic factors: fear, anxiety possibly evidenced by complaints of pain, self-focusing, guarding/distraction behaviors, restlessness, and autonomic responses (changes in vital signs).

Urinary elimination, altered patterns may be related to surgical diversion, tissue trauma, and postoperative edema possibly evidenced by loss of continence, changes in amount and character of urine, and urinary retention.

UROLITHIASIS (URINARY CALCULI) MS

Pain may be related to distention, trauma, and edema formation in sensitive tissue possibly evidenced by complaints (specify), guarding/distraction behaviors, self-focus, and autonomic responses (changes in vital signs).

Urinary elimination, altered patterns may be related to edema formation and irritation of ureteral and bladder tissues possibly evidenced by urgency, frequency, retention, and hematuria.

*Fluid volume deficit, potential** may be related to stimulation of renal-intestinal reflexes causing nausea, vomiting, and diarrhea; changes in urinary output; and decreased intake.

UTERINE BLEEDING, ABNORMAL GYN/MS

Anxiety (specify level) may be related to perceived change in health status and unknown etiol-

*Note: A potential diagnosis is not evidenced by signs and symptoms as the problem has not occurred and nursing interventions are directed at prevention.

ogy possibly evidenced by apprehension, uncertainty, fear of unspecified consequences, expressed concerns, and focus on self.

Activity intolerance may be related to imbalance between oxygen supply and demand/decreased oxygen-carrying capacity of blood (anemia) possibly evidenced by reports of fatigue/weakness.

UTERUS, RUPTURE OF, IN PREGNANCY — OB

Fluid volume deficit, (2) [active loss] may be related to excessive vascular losses possibly evidenced by hypotension, increased pulse rate, decreased venous filling, and decreased urine output.

Cardiac output, decreased may be related to decreased preload (hypovolemia) possibly evidenced by cold/clammy skin, decreased peripheral pulses, variations in hemodynamic readings, tachycardia, and cyanosis.

Pain may be related to tissue trauma and irritation of accumulating blood possibly evidenced by complaints (specify), guarding/distraction behaviors, self-focus, and autonomic responses (changes in vital signs).

Anxiety (specify level) may be related to threat of death of self/fetus possibly evidenced by fearful/scared affect, sympathetic stimulation, stated fear of unspecified consequences, and expressed concerns.

■ V

VAGINISMUS — GYN/CH

Pain may be related to muscle spasm and hyperesthesia of the nerve supply to vaginal mucous membrane possibly evidenced by complaints (specify), distraction behaviors, and self-focus.

Sexual dysfunction may be related to physical and/or psychologic alteration in function (severe spasms of vaginal muscles) possibly evidenced by verbalization of problem, inability to achieve desired satisfaction, and alteration in relationship with significant other.

VAGINITIS GYN/CH

Tissue integrity, impaired may be related to irritation/inflammation and mechanical trauma (scratching) of sensitive tissues possibly evidenced by damaged/destroyed tissue, presence of lesions.

Pain may be related to localized inflammation and tissue trauma possibly evidenced by complaints (specify), distraction behaviors, and self-focus.

Knowledge deficit [learning need] may be related to lack of information regarding hygienic and therapy needs and sexual behaviors/transmission of organisms possibly evidenced by statements of concern, questions, and misconceptions.

VARICES, ESOPHAGEAL

(Refer Also to Ulcer, Peptic) MS

Fluid volume deficit, (2) [active loss] may be related to excessive vascular loss, reduced intake, and gastric losses (vomiting) possibly evidenced by hypotension, tachycardia, decreased venous filling, and decreased/concentrated urine.

Anxiety (specify level)/Fear may be related to change in health status and threat of death possibly evidenced by increased tension/apprehension, sympathetic stimulation, restlessness, focus on self, and expressed concerns.

VARICOSE VEINS CH

Pain may be related to venous insufficiency and stasis possibly evidenced by complaints (specify).

Body image, disturbance may be related to change in structure (presence of enlarged, discolored tortuous superficial leg veins) possibly evidenced by hiding affected parts and negative feelings about body.

*Skin/Tissue integrity, impaired, potential** may be related to altered circulation/venous stasis and edema formation.

VENEREAL DISEASE

(Refer to Sexually Transmitted Disease) **CH**

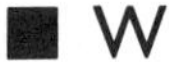 W

WILMS' TUMOR

(Refer Also to Cancer and Chemotherapy) **PED**

Anxiety (specify level)/Fear may be related to change in environment and interaction patterns with family members and threat of death with family transmission and contagion of concerns possibly evidenced by fearful/scared affect, distress, crying, insomnia, and sympathetic stimulation.

*Injury, potential for** may be related to nature of tumor (vascular, mushy with very thin covering) with increased danger of metastasis when manipulated.

Family processes, altered may be related to situational crisis of life-threatening illness possibly evidenced by a family system that has difficulty meeting physical, emotional, and spiritual needs of its members, and inability in dealing with traumatic experience effectively.

Diversional activity, deficit may be related to environmental lack of age-appropriate activity (including activity restrictions) and length of hospital-

---

*Note: A potential diagnosis is not evidenced by signs and symptoms as the problem has not occurred and nursing interventions are directed at prevention.

ization and treatment possibly evidenced by restlessness, crying, lethargy, and acting-out behavior.

WOUND, BULLET (DEPENDS ON SITE AND SPEED/CHARACTER OF BULLET) MS

Fluid volume deficit, potential* may be related to excessive vascular losses, altered intake/restrictions.

Pain may be related to destruction of tissue (including organ and musculoskeletal), surgical repair, and therapeutic interventions possibly evidenced by complaints (specify), guarding/distraction behaviors, self-focus, and autonomic responses (changes in vital signs).

Infection, potential for* may be related to tissue destruction and increased environmental exposure, invasive procedures, and decreased hemoglobin.

Post-trauma response, potential* may be related to nature of incident (catastrophic accident, assault, suicide attempt) and possible injury/death of other(s) involved.

---

*Note: A potential diagnosis is not evidenced by signs and symptoms as the problem has not occurred and nursing interventions are directed at prevention.

BIBLIOGRAPHY

Books

Berkow, R (ed): Merck Manual, ed 15. Merck & Co, Inc, Rahway, NJ, 1987.

Clinical Pocket Manual: Documentation. Nursing 88 Books, Springhouse Corp, Springhouse, PA, 1988.

Doenges, M and Moorhouse, M: Nurse's Pocket Guide: Nursing Diagnoses with Interventions, ed 2. FA Davis, Philadelphia, 1988.

Doenges, M, Kenty J, and Moorhouse, M: Maternal/Newborn Care Plans: Guidelines for Planning Patient Care. FA Davis, Philadelphia, 1988.

Doenges, M, Moorhouse, M, and Geissler, A: Nursing Care Plans: Guidelines for Planning Patient Care, ed 2. FA Davis, Philadelphia, 1989.

Doenges M, Townsend, M, and Moorhouse, M: Psychiatric Care Plans: Guidelines for Client Care. FA Davis, Philadelphia, 1989.

Fawcett, J. Analysis and Evaluation of Conceptual Models of Nursing, ed 2. FA Davis, Philadelphia, 1989.

Hazard, K and McCrea, T: Focus on the Nursing Process, Southwest Community Health Service, unpublished.

Kim, MJ, McFarland, GK, and McLane, AM (eds): Classification of Nursing Diagnoses. Proceedings of the Fifth National Conference. CV Mosby, St. Louis, 1984.

Lampe, SS: Focus Charting. Creative Nursing Management, Minneapolis, MN, 1986.

Moorhouse, M, Geissler, A, and Doenges, M: Critical Care Plans: Guidelines for Patient Care. FA Davis, Philadelphia, 1987.

Mumma, CM (ed): Rehabilitation Nursing: Concepts and Practice, A Core Curriculum, ed 2. Rehabilitation Nursing Foundation, Skokie, IL, 1987.

Nabors, F, Rocha, R, and Rafferty, F: Treatment Planning and Progress Notes, Austin, Texas, unpublished.

NANDA Taxonomy 1989. North American Nursing Diagnosis Association, St Louis, MO, 1989.

Nursing Science Quarterly: Theory, Research, and Practice. Williams & Wilkins, Baltimore, MD, February 1988.

Thomas, C (ed): Tabor's Cyclopedic Medical Dictionary, ed 16. FA Davis, Philadelphia, 1989.

Trieschman, AE, Whittaker, JK, and Brendtro, LK: The Other 23 Hours: Child Care Work with Emotionally Disturbed Children in a Therapeutic Milieu. Aidine de Gruyter, NY, 1969, pp 200–204.

Watson, J: Nursing: The Philosophy and Science of Caring. Colorado Associated University Press, Boulder, CO, 1985.

Watson, J: Nursing: Human Science and Human Care: A Theory of Nursing. Appleton-Century-Crofts, Norwalk, CT, 1985.

Articles

American Nurses' Association: Nursing: A social policy statement. Pub Code: NP-63 3SM 12/80, Kansas City, 1980.

American Nurses' Association: Standards of nursing practice. Pub Code: NO41 10M 1:77, Kansas City, 1973.

Eggland, ET: Charting: How and why to document your care daily—and fully. Nursing 88 18 (11):76–84, 1988.

Griffith-Kenney, JW and Christensen, PJ: Other frameworks and models. Nursing Process, Applications of Theories, Frameworks and Models, ed 2. CV Mosby, St. Louis, MO, 1986, pp 274–288.

Hanson, P: Focus charting—A new documentation tool. Coordinator, March 1986, pp 25–27.

Lampe, SS: Focus charting: Streamlining documentation. Nursing Management 16(7):43–46, 1985.

McCabe, BW: Evaluating the use of a focused data collection tool for the generation of nursing diagnoses: A replication study. Clinical Judgement and Decision-Making: The Future with Nursing Diagnosis. John Wiley & Sons, New York, 1987, pp 141–143.

Nicoll, LH (ed): Perspectives on nursing theory (Book Review). Image: Journal of Nursing Scholarship 18(4):183–184, 1986.

Schmieding, NJ: Putting Orlando's theory into practice. AJN 84(6):759–761, 1984.

Svanda, C: Two ways to sharpen your charting skills: Key words show what's important. RN December, 1986, pp 32–33.

INDEX

A page number in *italics* represents a figure; a page number followed by a "t" indicates a table. NANDA nursing diagnoses appear in *italics*.

KEY TO USE OF THIS MANUAL

This book is designed to aid the student as well as the clinician in care planning and documentation. In regard to the nursing process, this book is designed specifically to facilitate and validate the assessment and diagnosis stages of the process by means of the 300 disorders/health problems for which it provides associated nursing diagnostic statements.

1. *Data Collection:* The first step of the nursing process requires the collection of subjective and objective information from the patient (primary source) as well as secondary sources, for example, significant others, medical record, diagnostic testing, other health care providers (Chapter 3).

2. *Problem Identification:* If a particular disorder/health problem has been identified for the patient, reference to Section III enables the nurse to identify nursing diagnostic statements (which include etiologic labels and defining characteristics) commonly associated with the disorder/health problem. If the data collection tool suggests the presence of additional nursing diagnoses, the nurse is referred to one of several lists to determine these additional diagnoses. For data collection tools organized on a nursing model, the nurse may use either the Diagnostic Divisions list of nursing diagnoses (Table 3-1, p 32) or the list of nursing diagnoses grouped according to Gordon's Functional Health Patterns (inside back cover). For other types of assessment tools, the nurse is referred to the general

list of nursing diagnoses (Table 2-1, p 22). The nurse then validates each nursing diagnosis by adding the specific etiology ("related to" statements, and defining characteristics ("as evidenced by" statement) to create the individualized patient problem statement (Chapter 4).

3. *Planning:* The planning of care begins with goal setting (desired patient outcomes) that reflect measurable activities with specific/individualized time frames. This leads to the selection of appropriate interventions to achieve these goals for this patient (Chapter 4) and to the development of a complete, written plan of care. Section II provides seven prototype care plans, representing nearly every nursing specialty, which enables the reader to view the structure and content of a completed nursing care plan.

4. *Implementation:* The provision of a written plan facilitates implementation of care. Communication of this care provides for continuity and coordination of care between nurses and between nurses and other health team members. At this stage of the nursing process, charting becomes the critical means of coordinating care and of documenting the nursing actions called for under the care plan. Chapter 5 examines charting and establishes the context for the final stage of the nursing process, evaluation.

5. *Evaluation:* Assessment and documentation of nursing actions and patient response/condition lead to evaluation and provide for opportunity to make alterations and/or changes in care as identified. Throughout this process, careful documentation prevents duplication of work, provides a baseline for future comparisons, and records the nursing process and how it is applied to individual care. This also meets the needs of regulatory agencies, third-party payers, and legal requirements. (Chapter 5).